Table of Contents

Understanding Childhood Mental Disorders - 5

People, learn the art of communication - 8

Understanding Bipolar - 12

Understanding the Dynamics of Bipolar Disorder - 15

Combating Bipolar through Boot Camps - 18

Do I have Bipolar Disorder? - 20

Combating Childhood Depression - 23

Depression Triggers - 26

Fighting Depression - 29

Understanding Reactive Attachment Disorder - 33

RAD Causes - 35

Dealing with Attachment Issues in those with RAD - 38

Utilizing NeuroFeedback for RAD Diagnosis - 42

Understanding NeuroFeedback Treatments - 44

How to Help your Adopted Child Deal with RAD - 45

Strong Sitting -47

Attachment Therapists can help - 50

RAD is caused by a Lack of Love and Affection - 53

Utilizing EMDR as a Treatment - 55

Caring for Children with RAD - 58

RAD: In Adults - 60

Professional Writings about RAD - 63

How Strong Sitting can Help Children with RAD - 64

Craniosacral Therapy - 66

Tips on How to Handle RAD - 68

Dealing with RAD Patients who steal - 71

Attachment Therapy for RAD Children - 73

Breaking down the Barriers between you and your RAD Child - 78

Writings on RAD - 80

Identify RAD Symptoms - 81

Signs and Symptoms - 83

RAD Cool down Techniques - 86

Understanding how Eye Contact Affects RAD Children - 89

How to Help Children with Nonverbal Learning Disorders – 91

The Impact of a NLD - 99

ADHD Causes - 103

Important Information in Understanding ADHD - 105

Understanding the Differences between ODD and Normal Childhood Disobedience - 103

Symptoms of ODD - 105

Treating ODD - 108

Odd Treatments - 111

Remedies for ODD - 113

The Top Five Treatment Plans for Asperger's Syndrome - 117

Asperger's Syndrome Symptoms – 120

How PTSD Affects Sleep - 124

What are some of the Symptoms of PTSD? - 126

How Natural Disasters Spark PTSD - 129

Understanding Childhood Mental Disorders

Childhood disorders, which are also referred to as developmental or learning disorders, are certain types of mental illnesses that are diagnosed in children during their earliest years. Though, at times, certain adults may also exhibit signs of similar mental illnesses, the symptoms begin to be apparent during a child's formative years and are hence, termed as childhood disorders.

In fact, a recent study has revealed that, in the United States alone, almost 12 million children suffer from mood disorders of one kind or another and only one in every five of these children ever receive the proper treatment. Adults, who suffer from such disruptive mental health issues, will cause their children to exhibit signs of mood disorders.

There is a popular saying that says that the child years of a person are the best, but, this is not always the case. A child can be overtly exposed to a lot of emotional issues that will result in tremendous stress and strain, if they are not tackled properly. This compels them to go through painful situations almost as much as – and sometimes more than - an adult. These situations will have an everlasting impact on the immature mindset of the children, leaving them temporally mentally disoriented and, at times, permanently damaged.

Now, let's look into various types of mood disorders and mental illness that are generally observed amongst children.

- *Depression*: This is one of the most common types of mental illnesses that are found in children. In fact, in the Unites States alone, there are as many as six million children who are suffering from depression. The common symptoms include a sense of sadness and helplessness, extreme fatigue, and a low and fragile self-esteem with a lack of ability to express emotions and feelings.
- Another very common type of mental disorder is *Attention Deficit Disorder* (ADD) which is also called *Attention Deficit Hyperactivity Disorder* (ADHD). About 10 percent of American children are suffering from this mental illness which is associated with the lack of an ability to concentrate on and learn anything with a propensity of hyperactivity. Usually, children younger than the age of 7 develop this illness.
- *Reactive Attachment Disorder* (RAD) is another common form of mental illness that is found in children. The main reason behind this comes from continuous negligence, abuse, and violence during, the child's younger years. This results in an inability to grow and develop healthy relationships, during the subsequent stages of life.
- *Conduct Disorder* (CD) is the most common type of mental illness that is found in children. Though certain experts term this ailment as simple rebellion or juvenile delinquency - that is far from reality. In fact, this is the direct result of various mood disorders that have gone unnoticed or undiagnosed.

Causes of Childhood Disorders

One of the major reasons for childhood mental disorders is the troubled marriage of their parents and their subsequent separation. Children of separated couples have a higher propensity of developing these disorders, as the effects of separation or troubled relation between their parents, take a severe toll on their infantile mindset. These hapless children are usually found to be suffering from trauma or anxiety disorder. This stops them from developing relationships and they will begin to suffer from a phobia; sometimes, they will not even be able to spend a night at a friend's or relative's house, unless they are accompanied by a relative or either of their parents.

Parents, learn the art of communication

During the infantile – puberty stages, the rate of growth seems to fly by and suddenly, your tiny toddler, who was playing with toys the other day, has grown and wants to go out with friends to have fun. Everything seems to happen in a blink of an eye. The child's development and growth is that fast and therefore, it becomes the responsibility of the parent/s to assess every stage of this development – physically, as well as, intellectually, so that the child can be prepared to have a great life, as an adult.

Since spotting cognitive or intellectual changes in a child's brain is not that easy, you can gauge these changes by observing the way that the child sees and uses new things at various stages during the growth period. It's important for your child and this is why child-parent interaction is imperative.

While you can easily understand the physical growth of your child, in order to evaluate the intellectual growth, better communication with your child is needed. Ask certain questions and the answers that you get will provide you with an insight into the behavior and developmental changes that are taking place in your child's mind. To help you with this, the following are some tips you can learn from -

How can I Gauge My Child's Psychology?

In order to assess the cognitive growth of your child, you need to be aware about certain things about them. For instance, you have to be careful about things that may make your child angry. The things that make the child feel embarrassed or feel fear should be clear to you, so that you can understand what makes them tick. To understand all of this, you have to communicate with your child, as much as possible. Since children's mind are far more sensitive than that of the adults, you need to know how you can better communicate with them.

Finding out information about your child's favorite color or the shade that s/he wants for his or her room can help you get closer to them. You can also ask your child about their favorite subject in school and try to figure out why they enjoy that subject. Knowing about the kind of peer group that s/he mingles with and whom your kid idolizes can also give you understanding about the cognitive development that is taking place in their mind. Gathering these details is important, because from these, you can analyze the behavioral patterns and intellectual levels of your child's mind.

Consider asking your kid about how s/he feels when interacting with others. Inquiring about his or her favorite TV shows and books are also some good questions to ask. You can also ask your child about the way that s/he likes to spend the holidays or weekends, and who, outside of the immediate family, s/he thinks has played a crucial role in their life. Also, you can ask them about what changes that they would like to see occur in you or your family's life. These kinds of questions will not only help you assess the mental growth of your child, but, they will draw you closer to your child.

In addition to these, there are a few more details that you can find out about your child, as you endeavor to assess his or her cognitive growth at various ages. A few of these are listed below:

- The accomplishments that make your child feel proud
- Their biggest disappointments in life
- What is their most cherished gift?
- When does s/he like to do his homework?
- How does s/he feel at home?

Bipolar Disorder

Understanding Bipolar

What is bipolar disorder?

To start out with, we should try to understand what bipolar disorder actually is. Clinically speaking, it is the psychosomatic diagnosis for various types of mental disorders, in which patients suffer from a variety of disruptive and collaborative mood swings. Bipolar disorder is also referred to as bipolar affective disorder.

The ailment is generally associated with a hyperactive state of mind which is commonly termed as mania. In general, bipolar disorder is associated with one or multiple bouts of elevated and irritable levels of energy, arousal, or moods that are opposing toward one another. However, having this disorder, along with visible episodes of a depressive mental state is also quite common.

Due to prolonged research, which has been conducted on patients of bipolar disorder and their mental state, we can understand bipolar disorder more and learn important facts about it. The ailment does not have any relations, whatsoever, with the highs and lows of our daily life. The causes of this ailment are far deeper rooted. The ailment tends to cause severe and long lasting damage to relationships, career, and performance on professional and academic fronts. Fortunately, the ailment is very much treatable, if found early enough and more importantly, a proper diagnosis will speed up recovery and help the patient to get back to their normal life.

Symptoms of Bipolar Disorder

Some of the most common symptoms of this disorder are discussed in greater depth in the following segment. Symptoms usually begin show through any of the following mannerisms or belief systems -

- A fairly elevated state of mental, as well as, frequent physical activities

- Frequent bouts of expansive behavior and abnormal exaggeration of optimism

- An overstated sense of self importance

- Irritating and often aggressive behavior

- Sleeplessness that does not cause any fatigue

- Difficulty in their thought process, with the inability of proper judgment

- Excessively rapid rate of speech and the patient often keeps on talking continuously and behave rather recklessly

- Patients of bipolar disorder often manifest inappropriate sexual behaviors

- Occasional occurrences of hallucinations and delusions are observed in certain patients

- Occasional bouts of depression and prolonged period of unreasonable sadness during which, the patients resort to sobbing for hardly any – or no - reason at all

- Rapid mood swings when the patient remains irritated, anxious, and worried, they will also constantly agitating people around him or her

- Showing signs of depression accompanied by prolonged phase of unreasonable sadness, apathy, and lethargy

- Lack of interest in normal activities or will have relationships, but lack the zeal to live, often accompanied by thoughts of death and sometimes, an urge to commit suicide

- Having constant nightmares and wetting bed during night

- Noticeable change of eating habits and a consistent desire for a lot of sweets and carbohydrates

- Inability to control anger with the rage lasting for hours, even, days

- Change in patterns of sleep with the patient sleeping too much or not sleeping at all.

Causes of Bipolar Disorder

Though the exact cause of Bipolar Disorder could not be ascertained, in some cases, there is a substantial genetic contribution, while in other cases, certain environmental influences are said to be responsible for the ailment.

Understanding the Dynamics of Bipolar Disorder

Lately, Bipolar disorder has become one of the most common psychological ailments that children are being diagnosed with. The reason behind this is a wide range of socio-economic problems which are plaguing modern society. Children are easily falling prey to these problems and psychologists are complaining about the alarming rise in the number of children who are suffering from bipolar disorder symptoms. Due to this, you may hear about campaigns that are organized from time to time. These campaigns are designed for pharmaceutical marketing, as well as, to spread awareness about this mental disorder and its treatment. However, there are still several misconceptions which people may fall prey to about this mental health issue. This is because people still don't know much about it and its treatment. In order to get rid of some of the most common myths, a few truths about bipolar disorder will be discussed here.

Bipolar Disorder facts

As are most mental disorders, Bipolar disorder is a severe mental condition. However, its severity cannot be said to be more than any other type of mental disorders. A person who is suffering from a mental disorder cannot be considered crazy or insane. It only means that the person is having a hard time and these hard times are negatively affecting the way that s/he lives his/her life. In the absence of timely treatment, these mental conditions can lead to a situation of distress and lead to a wide array of complications and will affect interpersonal relationships.

A type of mood disorder

Bipolar disorder is a kind of mood disorder and to describe it accurately, its old name of 'manic depression' was changed to bipolar disorder. The mood of a person generally swings between that of episodes of depression and manic.

Psychotherapy to treat the signs of bipolar disorder

A lot of people and medical professionals believe that psychotherapy cannot help patients with this kind of mental disorder. However, the fact is that, psychotherapy can prove beneficial in the treatment of bipolar disorder. With the help of psychotherapy, a person can be trained to deal with the feelings of depressive or manic episodes.

Psychotherapy helps a patient to lead his life with the disorder without getting them stressed out or upset. Many people who are diagnosed with this mental ailment don't go for psychotherapy when they are first diagnosed, thus, aggravating the situation further. However, the fact is it can prove highly beneficial for the patients who have been diagnosed; it can help them in their process toward healing.

Patients need to take medications as prescribed

There are some people who stop taking medications because they think they are feeling well and hence, in their mind, there is no longer any need to continue their medication. This is a common misconception that affects the patients severely. Patients with bipolar disorder need to take their medication as recommended, even when he or she feels good.

Needs proper diagnosis

More often than not, bipolar disorder is confused with clinical depression because depression is one of the primary symptoms of this mental issue. About 25% people with this disorder are, at first, misdiagnosed with depression. The reason behind this is that the majority of people approach their primary health care specialists for diagnosis of depression and the primary medical healthcare providers do not always ask the sufficient questions which would help them to understand whether it is a case of common depression or a graver case of bipolar disorder. However, the same can be the case with mental health professionals, as well. Due to an incorrect initial diagnosis, the patient is prescribed antidepressants, which is not a treatment for bipolar disorder.

In fact, the wrong treatment can lead to complications in the person. So it's better that you go for a proper diagnosis. For instance, if you experience an episode of heightened energy without any specific reason, then, you should discuss it with a mental health expert.

Combating Bipolar through Boot Camps

If your child is suffering from Bipolar Disorder that is surely not something that you would be very elated about. Again, this is something that should not be an absolute heart break for you. In fact, you should thank your lucky stars that you know what actually is wrong with your child. You will find a lot of kids with symptoms of Bipolar Disorder and you will, also, find out that their parents are somewhat relieved that, at least, they know how they can proceed in dealing with their children who have symptoms of BD.

A lot of treatment methodologies have been innovated to deal with children who have Bipolar Disorder symptoms. One of them is the Juvenile boot camps. Though, initially, the concept of boot camps were to deal with prisoners and acted more as detention camps than anything else, to patients of Bipolar Disorder, these boot camps have become like rehabs where their ailments are taken into account and acted upon. They also act as intervention camps for these children. However, depending upon the gravity of the situation and severity of the ailment, certain boot camps may use various ruthless, challenging, and demanding methods of treatment that are even enforced through a lot of verbal hostilities and physically challenging designs under the supervision of drill sergeants, you may not want to send your child there. All of these camps are immaculately designed to "intervene and break" the very spirit of the teenagers who are suffering from Bipolar Disorder.

The entire idea is to use the treatment curriculum that would assist these children in rebuilding their self esteem via the basis of discipline and respect. However, the children suffering from Bipolar Disorder symptoms should only be sent to these boot camps when things begin to spiral out of controlling and are heading toward the worst case scenario. Only when these people become manic should they be subjected to these harsh forms of treatment as this remains the only way to deal with the situation.

Another school of thought says that this is not the right way to deal with Bipolar Disorder. This is because of the harsh treatment at these camps, at times, may impart a sense of bad behavior for these children even, after they come out of their ailment. That is why, though boot camps, at times, are handy when dealing with this disorder, when a patient leaves, the camp may leave a permanent effect on the psyche of the patient. This could further affect their Bipolar Disorder.

Therefore, it is better to employ the help of a counselor or a psychiatrist who can treat these patients far better and with more empathy and consideration for the patient.

Do I have Bipolar Disorder?

Bipolar disorder, which is also called bipolar affective disorder, is a specific psychiatric condition of mind that results in mood disorders which lead to highly disruptive mood swings. Here are some of the most prominent symptoms, which should be examined when trying to figure out if the patient is suffering from Bipolar disorder. These are almost unmistakable signs of Bipolar Disorder, on which the basis of the treatment is conducted.

Mania: Occasional signs of extreme energy and sudden bouts of excessive excitement for little or no reason. At times, such outbursts of energy are accompanied by loss of sleep for a prolonged period. Arguments which are triggered by apparently soft and innocent queries are also regarded as some of the most common symptoms of Bipolar Disorder.

Hypomania: The signs of Hypomania are exactly the same as that of Mania but, only in a milder form. Whether a patient of Bipolar disorder shows signs of Mania or Hypomania entirely depend upon the extent of seriousness of the ailment of the individual in question.

Depression: A patient of Bipolar disorder may, at times, exhibit extreme forms of depression. This state of mind is associated with acute sadness for little or no reason. During this period, the patient may resort to continuous crying with a tendency of isolation from family members and friends. These Bipolar Disorder symptoms are generally associated with a suicidal tendency, backed by a loss of interest towards life. This is a dangerous phase during which the patient is needed to be kept under strict vigil.

Mixed Symptoms: This is again one of those typical symptoms of Bipolar Disorder in which the patient shows severe depression and a saddened mood but, is devoid of lethargy, unlike the typical signs of depression. Interestingly, while the patient continues to suffer from depression, the person will also have enough energy to take a sprint! This is often associated with disturbed appetite and patterns of sleeping. However, in most cases, Bipolar Disorder does not show this particular symptom and hence, this is one of the less obvious symptoms of Bipolar Disorder.

Basically, there are two types of Bipolar Disorder – Variety I and Variety II. The symptoms of Bipolar disorder generally vary depending upon the two varieties. While Bipolar Disorder I symptoms include manic and at times, have mixed episodes, which may last for as many as 7 to 10 days at a time, symptoms of the other variety are vastly different. Patients of Bipolar Disorder II generally show bouts of mild to severe depression that may, at times, be associated with hypomania. This implies that patients of Bipolar Disorder II do not show any extreme manic behavioral symptoms except for hypomania, which is a far less fatal manic episode.

Both of the two varieties of Bipolar Disorder are easily curable if they are diagnosed at an early stage. However, patients who are addicted to substances develop a higher risk factor if suffering from Bipolar Disorder and need to be immediately taken to rehabilitation centers for a prolonged treatment that may last for months to years, depending upon the extent of addiction.

Childhood Depression

Combating Childhood Depression

Studies, which were conducted by experts over a considerable period of time, have revealed that depression, in almost five percent of all cases; occur before the age of 12. Naturally, the tender and immature mindsets of the affected children get devastated, which tends to leave a horrifying impact on their families.

In a lot of cases, depression, which apparently seems to have no drastic effect on the affected kid, often gets unnoticed or under-diagnosed, which can leave a disastrous effect on the child in question. Now, you may be wondering how you will notice that your child is suffering from depression. Let us get right into that. The symptoms of depression generally include:

- A constant feeling of frustration, sadness, and loss of self-importance

- Occurrence of certain physical complications, which include headaches, pain, stiffness in muscles, stomach related problems, excessive tiredness, and lethargy

- A feat of facing anything and a tendency of running away from everything

- Sudden bouts of anger which accompanies shouting, irritation, and sobbing for hardly any – or no reason at all

- A complete listlessness in their outlook and attitude, coupled by a sudden lack of interest in things which used to generate a lot of pleasure in their life

- Tendency of isolating from the society that is backed by lack of ability to properly communicate with others;

- Too much sensitivity to failure or rejection marked by some reckless attitudes

- Too much sleep or a lack of sleep

- Thoughts of committing suicide and an intense sense of inferiority complex

Expert Opinions

Experts believe that childhood depression is often caused by the following issues -

- Children with a trouble childhood due to a disturbed family can develop symptoms of depression

- Children, who are subjected to excessive stress and strain, can suffer from nervous breakdown which can lead to depression

- Children, who see death of either of their parents or both of them in early childhood, have a propensity of developing depression

- Depression in children can also result from any chronic illness which may impart a sense of frustration in them when they see others of the same age leading a normal, gleeful, and healthy life.

- Constant abuse and lack of affection during their childhood days can result in depression in children

The first and foremost thing that the parents of a child who is suffering from depression should remember that the ailment is very much curable. They need to be optimistic and should never lose hope. Only then, will they be able to take care of their child properly. There are various types of treatment available which can help to take care of depression. Treatments include various types of medications, short-term psychotherapy courses, or a method which employs both of the processes.

Depending upon the severity of the ailment, children with depression can either be treated at home or can be admitted in certain schools for a more compact, cohesive, and holistic treatment. The treatment that is conducted is perfectly designed to assist the child in understanding and expressing their feelings of frustration and agony in a safe and a proper manner. Also, their families will benefit from these treatments by learning the ways that they can cope with these kids suffering from depression. The only thing that is needed is to have an early detection and then, appropriate steps can be taken.

Depression Triggers

Typically, there are a number of different factors which can trigger depression in any person. These can be a mix of biological, psychological, genetic, and environmental factors. In some medical theories, one of the causes of depression is suggested to be the imbalance of neurotransmitters in brain.

Neurotransmitters are a kind of chemical that assists the brain cells in their communication with one another. However, due to the lack of concrete proofs, this theory cannot be accepted wholeheartedly.

According to scientists, some depression can be hereditary and some forms may even occur without a family history. In order to better indentify the symptoms of depression, certain genes, which are likely to make some people depression prone, are currently being researched. A few results of this study show that depression can take place in a person when several genes act together in response to environmental - or other - changes. Though it is believed that depressive episodes can occur in a person without any particular reason, there are some situations which can lead to its occurrence.

To in order to delve deeper into this subject matter, Magnetic Resonance Imaging (MRI) – which is a brain imaging technology – has been used. The results of this technology show that the brain of a person with depression looks different from that of a normal person. Certain parts of the brain, which are associated with sleep, appetite, thinking, behaviors, and mood, tend to look different in the person who struggles with depression. But the problem is that this technology is also unable to trace the actual causes of depression.

However, there are some symptoms which can be identify the cause of depression in any individual person. A few of such symptoms are being listed below:

Different Possible Symptoms of Depression

• Lack of concentration

• Tendency to feel sad

• Inability to take right decisions

• Lack of problem-solving skills

• Lack of hope for bright future

• Fear of failure

• Tendency to feel guilty or despair

• Negative outlook about self and performance

• Feeling of dissatisfaction over things

• Tendency to over-criticize one own self for seeming mistakes or weaknesses

- Feeling of being punished
- Suicidal thoughts
- Low self esteem
- Feeling of irritation and annoyance
- Energy loss
- Unsatisfied sex life and relationship
- Feelings of unattractiveness
- Less control over tears or inability to cry
- Fast weight loss or gain
- Inability to handle projects
- Changes in eating and sleeping habits
- Worries related to physical problems, pains, and aches

These are some of the common causes of depression which can be found in both men and women. If these tendencies are not checked on time, a person can become victim of this ailment. In order to avoid this situation, it's important to fight depression. Medical help, regular exercise, and proper nutrition are a must in order to maintain the mental health. In addition, the person needs to express his or her feelings well. He or she should try to find out the problem areas which are causing depressing feelings in him/her, though, the person should try not to dwell on them. Also, the person should always look at the positive side of life, instead of thinking about the negatives.

Fighting Depression

While Depression is not considered a life threatening ailment, it is, by all means, a potentially lethal one, considering the fact that it takes a heavy toll on the social, as well as, the professional life of an individual. Hence, an individual should always be subjected to a proper treatment upon showing even the slightest signs of depression. This prevents the situation from spiraling out of hand.

However, that does not mean that people who may experience depressed feelings at times should be subjected to treatment but, there are certain alarming depression symptoms that, if noticed, should be taken care of.

The effects of depression vary from person to person. While in some, there is only the need of psychological treatment, others may have deep rooted problems which demand thorough medication which will need to be taken for a prolonged period, along with deep psychological treatment.

Generally speaking, depression symptoms include:

- Sudden loss of pleasure and interest in things and subjects that the individual generally enjoys

- Lack of sleep or too much sleep

- A sense of worthlessness or of remorse, frustration or guilt

- Inability to make wise decisions and a disturbed thought process, along with a severe lack of concentration

Depending upon the severity of these depression effects, the mode of treatment is decided. Drugs that are most commonly used to treat depression are anti-depressants, which are composed to reduce or relieve the effects and signs of depression.

Generally, the following types of anti-depressants are used for treatment. With each of these medicines being unique in composition, they have their own method of arresting the signs of depression.

Serotonin Reuptake Inhibitors (SSRIs):

The use of this particular anti-depressant stops the nerve cells from reabsorbing the neurotransmitter serotonin after releasing it. This helps the serotonin to work continuously and actively.

Fluoxetine and Sertraline are two of most commonly used SSRIs in the treatment of depression.

Other types of anti - depressants that are often prescribed are Norepinephrine Reuptake Inhibitors (SNRI) and Selective Serotonin Norepinephrine Reuptake Inhibitors (SSNRI).

The SNRIs that are most often used include, Duloxetine and Venlafaxine. Other types and classes of anti-depressants are also used in treating depression; however, which medicine one is prescribed, depends upon the signs and symptoms that are being exhibited by the patient. It is generally believed that virtually all types of anti-depressants have a wide variety of side effects attached to them. That is why, it is much better to resort to psychological treatment instead of administering any drugs.

Psychological treatment that a depressed individual is generally subjected to includes:

- **Cognitive Behavior Therapy** or CBT: It is believed to be the most effective way of treating depression. CBT is a controlled curriculum that is designed to restructure the feelings of the patients by restructuring the thoughts. It also helps the patient to think positively and have affirmative views toward their life.

- **Interpersonal Therapy** or IPT: This particular method of treating depression is applied if the patient gets easily influenced and depressed by comments or criticisms that other people make toward them. This therapy helps people to think positively and to shrug off the effects of these comments. It also teaches them to use those comments in a positive way for self-development.

- **Family Therapy**: This is designed to teach friends and family members to understand depression symptoms and help a depressed friend or a member of their family come out of the depression.

Reactive Attachment Disorder

Understanding Reactive Attachment Disorder

Reactive attachment disorder (RAD) is commonly found in infants and children who don't have a healthy relationship with their parents - or other close relatives. Children, who have been neglected or abused from a young age - and children, who were orphans - generally tend to develop this psychological issue. The situation continues to develop the longer that a child is deprived of his or her basic needs of comfort, affection, and nurturing. As a result of this, the brain development of the child gets affected, which further hinders his or her ability to build healthy relationships. Though this mental health disease is a lifelong condition, it can be treated to help children understand how they can enter into a healthy relationship with their parents and caregivers.

According to medical experts, it's the tendency of each individual to make conclusions about his or her situations, experiences, and people that they are around. All this is done with the help of sense organs which align these experiences. For instance, a particular smell or sound will sometimes trigger an individual's memory with certain time or place. When this happens, an individual is reminded of the original situation and also of his or her reaction to that. This is a continuous process as every individual links his or her past conclusions with current experiences. If the past is not a pleasant one, this process may stop, halt, or get frozen. If this process gets interrupted because of an abusive past of the individual, then it leads to RAD frozen conclusions.

Dr. Joanne May has pointed out that there are seven frozen conclusions of RAD, which are accepted by the children who suffer from reactive attachment disorder. These are as following -

Reactive Attachment Disorder Frozen Conclusions

- I am getting such treatment because I am bad or evil
- I need to be in control if I want to survive
- I can never do anything right
- I deserve hatred from the ones around me
- People around me deserve my hatred
- I should not trust adults or those in authority because it might not be safe for me
- I am evil and/or bad and my behavior is my signature that clearly states who I am

If you think your child is having reactive attachment disorder, you should take him or her to your family physician or any general practitioner for treatment. During treatment, parents and caregivers of the affected child need to be present. Treatment for this kind of mental illness generally includes periodic psychological counseling and a thorough course of medication, the extent of which varies depending upon the severity of the ailment. Other than this, there are a few other methods which are options that you may take in your pursuit of getting RAD treatment.

RAD Causes

Reactive Attachment Disorder (RAD) can be described as a severe and relatively rare type of a mental disorder that generally affects children. The ailment is associated with obvious disturbed and developmentally improper ways of establishing relations in various social contexts. Now, what really are the causes of Reactive Attachment Disorder? According to the experts, there are a number of reasons behind RAD and they need to be ascertained accurately in order to receive effective RAD treatment.

Broadly speaking, the following can be termed as the principle Reactive Attachment Disorder causes.

- In a lot of cases, drugs or other types of substance abuse including, alcoholism are believed to be amongst the most commonly found causes of Reactive Attachment Disorder
- Defective birth procedures and trauma experienced during birth is also said to be one of the greatest causes for Reactive Attachment Disorder

- In young women, unwanted pregnancy, at times, will give rise to Reactive Attachment Disorder
- Another main causes of Reactive Attachment Disorder is severe abuse, be it, sexual, physical, or emotional, at the very earliest stage of life, notably within the first three years
- Separation from parents, especially the mother right from the time of birth is believed to be one of the most prominent RAD causes
- Children who are being brought up in highly chaotic and disturbing family environment may at times show symptoms of RAD.
- Children who are constantly abused or physically and emotionally neglected generally fall prey to RAD
- Unsympathetic and inconsistent way of parenting is also believed to be one of the reasons behind RAD
- If a child is being constantly compelled to change homes at early stages of life at times may develop symptoms of Reactive Attachment Disorder
- Overindulging parenting is also believed to be one of the main reasons behind RAD
- Taking care of the child inadequately and improperly sometimes result in RAD
- If the child is being taken care of by multiple care givers, that may cause reasons behind Reactive Attachment Disorder
- Failed or improper adoption is one of the most prominent Reactive Attachment Disorder causes
- If the child is frequently moved from one location to another resulting in a drastic and repeated change in the foster care system that may result in development of Reactive Attachment Disorder
- If the child goes through a traumatic experience for a considerable time that will surely result in

development of RAD symptoms as the fallout of the incident
- If there is a case of a painful illness that has been left undiagnosed and hence is causing immense and prolonged physical pain, that may give rise to Reactive Attachment Disorder subsequently.
- Cases of maternal alcohol or substance abuse is said to be one of the principle Reactive Attachment Disorder causes
- Maternal depression when the child is young, may at times affect the child's psyche giving rise to symptoms of Reactive Attachment Disorder
- If there is deficit of attunement between the mother and her child for a prolonged period starting immediately after the child's birth that will result in Reactive Attachment Disorder subsequently.
- Young and inexperienced mothers who are not skilled in parenting obviously results in development of Reactive Attachment Disorder symptoms in the child.

Dealing with Attachment Issues in people with RAD

There is a difference between reactive attachment disorder (RAD) and attachment issues. A child is most likely to feel a lot of mental stress if he is shifted from one home to another and if he is taken to new parents. He will face attachment issues, even if the previous surroundings and relations were abusive. The child has to accept the new arrangement, irrespective of whether the new home and surroundings are better or worse than the previous one. This exerts a lot of strain on their psyche resulting in the development of RAD in certain cases.

According to medical experts, even if a child is not diagnosed with RAD attachment issues, he may take one year or more to get familiar with the new family where he has been shifted and its members. Initially, there can be signs of reluctance or hesitation, which is a normal, and the quicker the new parents and other family members understand this, it is easier for them to adopt the child and for the child to accept them. This mutual understanding helps in better bonding between the child and the parents and this helps the child to adjust to the new situation quickly. Moreover, the transition of the child gets easier and effortless.

Attachment issues may result from a number of factors. Most often than not, children who are either adopted or brought up in foster systems are found to face RAD attachment problems. However, this condition can also be witnessed in biologically intact families.

Symptoms of Reactive Attachment Disorder

Birth to 6 Months

- Frequent shouting and/ or social withdrawal
- Resisting physical touch, at times, touch can lead to violent reaction from the child
- Efforts to soothe one own self through some repetitive acts
- Showing resistance to comforting gestures shown by the caregivers

Result:

If the issues of attachment in RAD children are not addressed at this age, he may develop a negative self-identity, a feeling of rage, and several learning, as well as behavioral, problems.

6 to 10 Months

- Self-soothing, proved by rocking
- Early signs of maturity
- Absence of stranger anxiety
- Self reliance

10 to 18 Months

- An acute feeling of separation
- Showing no interest in exploring the world
- Throwing out frustration in the form of aggressive behavior

15 to 24 Months

- Hyper vigilant
- Clingy
- Reserved
- Inability to integrate dependence and independence
- Transition issues or difficulty in adapting to sudden changes

Result:

If these reactive attachment disorder issues are not corrected at an early age, then, the feeling of separation anxiety may aggravate further, which will cause troubles when he starts going to school. Also, these complications at such a tender age can also cause a feeling of failure or frustration in the child, leading to anger, low self esteem, and extreme anxiety.

24 to 36 Months

- Hyper vigilance
- Tendency to cling
- Difficulty in adjusting to changing situations
- Failure to connect emotionally

If attachment issues persist in a child, even, when his elementary education starts, they are quite likely to become stronger and in some cases, it may turn into an attachment disorder. A child identified with reactive attachment disorder does not trust the people in authority and considers them to be nasty, exploitative, and unpredictable. The child may not show through his outward behavior that he is feeling responsible for the thing that has happened, but he may blame himself secretly for everything bad that has taken place.

Children facing attachment disorder conditions are good at manipulating things and mastering skills which are important for their survival. But, at the same time, these conditions can also be a source of immense stress for the family members. These conditions may lead to unfavorable consequences if not tackled properly. Hence, it's important to provide RAD treatment to the affected children on time for positive results.

Utilizing Neurofeedback for RAD Diagnosis

The symptoms of an attachment issue or reactive attachment disorder (RAD) are commonly found in orphaned or adopted children. In addition to this, several not-too-friendly situations of life can also be the cause of this mental health condition in children. However, it should be noted that RAD can occur even in a child who is with his family and is neither adopted nor orphaned. Not many people know much about this mental condition and hence, it becomes important to get proper diagnosis of RAD and learn about its symptoms and treatment procedures.

According to medical health experts, the signs of attachment disorder are frequent mood swings, behavioral changes and withdrawal from social relationships. These happen when a child fails to establish relationship with his primary caregivers such as mother and other close ones in the family in his early childhood period. This mental condition can occur in a child during his early developmental stages such as 2 to 6 years. The symptoms develop as the child grows and faces difficulty in adjusting to social environments, conforming to accepted behavioral patterns, etc.

Since these symptoms may take years to grow and become obvious to the eyes of the parents and others, it becomes difficult to diagnose this disease. With rising demands for social interactions and performance issues in school, the problem even gets worse. However, thanks to awareness and a lot of information available from various sources, today the symptoms are recognizable pretty early. Some symptoms which are pretty prominent and easily recognizable include tendency to remain unattached with primary caregivers, mood swings, anxiety, stress, etc. On the basis of these and other symptoms which are also clinically tested, a child with this kind of disorder can now be offered useful treatment at an early stage. Currently, neurofeedback in RAD treatment is proving to be quite helpful.

Understanding Neurofeedback Treatments

RAD is a mental condition related to brain and neurofeedback is one of the strongest tools that can be used for the brain. That is why, more and more attachment therapists are going for neurofeedback in RAD treatment. With the help of this treatment, children learn to control their anger, anxiety and stress under different situations.

Basically, neurofeedback in RAD treatment helps children to control their brain activity. It deals with those parts of the brain which help human beings to stay calm. With RAD neurofeedback treatment, a RAD patient learns to control his emotions. According to mental health experts, the victims of attachment issues find difficulty in self-regulation and lack the ability to calm down. Besides, RAD patients also fail to handle emotions and are likely to face several other developmental problems that plague the natural course of their life. Neurofeedback can prove beneficial for a RAD patient on all these fronts. Also, the use of neurofeedback in RAD treatment as an alternative to medications can help patients with RAD symptoms to decrease or get rid of drugs as their brains gain stability.

How to Help your Adopted Child Deal with RAD

Adopted children, especially, the ones who are adopted later in their life, are most likely to develop reactive attachment disorder symptoms. Parenting these children can be a challenging task because these children don't want to build any attachment with their primary caregivers. Hence, in such a situation, it becomes absolutely essential to bring certain changes in one's own parenting style. For help, you can search through some special content on the internet and buy books and DVDs, which offer extensive information on tackling reactive attachment disorder (RAD) patients.

For help, you can go through the book called <u>When Love is Not Enough</u> by Nancy Thomas. The book serves as a useful source of information on how to deal with RAD in adopted children. The book's content can be extremely helpful because the author herself has parented RAD children for a long period of time and all the information that she has penned down is inspired from her own practical experiences.

First of all, you need to identify the reactive attachment disorder symptoms in your child. This can be done by observing his behavior at different stages of his life. To know whether your child feels unattached towards the members of your family and is suffering from RAD symptoms, you need to closely observe his behavior at various ages. Some of his behaviors may be – taking whatever things he encounters and wants (between 1 and 3 years of age), stop taking things that he encounters and wants simply because he is afraid that his parents would kill him (between 3 and 5 years of age), not taking things that he sees and desires to have simply because he feels his parents will be upset (between 5 and 9 years of age), and showing no interest in a thing even when he sees and likes it because he may not feel comfortable about it (between 9 and 11 years of age), etc.

Other than this, if you notice that your child avoids eye contact, throws excessive tantrums, or resist hugs and kisses from you, then, you may have reason to believe that s/he is showing reactive attachment disorder symptoms. Also, age – regression techniques, such as, not acting his age, can also be an indication of RAD. For instance, if you give your 12 year old child something that he asked for and he behaves like a 2 or 3 year old in response, then, this may be a sign of RAD.

In order to deal with these symptoms of RAD in your child, you need to take help of an experienced child's therapist who possesses significant knowledge in the field of various attachment therapies. Additionally, since these children exhibit the tendency of being in power, parents need to show them the right direction. If your child also shows this tendency, it becomes your responsibility to take him to the right direction. For this, you can learn about the techniques mentioned in the book by Nancy Thomas.

Being a parent of the child with reactive attachment disorder symptoms, you need to practice patience and positivity. Make sure that your expectations are realistic. If you do these, you will get enough courage and hope to build a strong relationship with your child.

Strong Sitting

A child suffering from reactive attachment disorder (RAD) may not be able to focus on things around him. His brain seems to race 100 miles an hour without any break. Due to this, the child may find difficulty in concentrating on chores or problem-solving tasks. To improve this situation, the child must be given RAD treatment and an ideal treatment of RAD is strong sitting. Strong sitting for RAD treatment can help children develop patience and self-control. If a child is quiet both physically and emotionally, strong stilling will help the child perform the tasks well.

If your kid cannot stay dry, you can give him a rubber-backed rug for this purpose and once he is done with his strong sitting for RAD treatment, he can clean that. Make sure to choose a safe and comfortable spot for your child where he will be doing this. The place should not be far from your view. There should not be any scope for distractions. Some people suggest their children to strong sit just close to the bedroom door, so that they can be easily monitored from outside while doing a daily household job. Along with this, there are certain other factors that need your close attention while your child is doing strong sitting.

Points to remember while the child is strong sitting for RAD treatment

- Make sure your child's legs are folded in Indian style and he sits with his head and back straight. He can keep his hands on his lap, thighs or even on the floor.
- RAD strong sitting can be little difficult for the child at the beginning because he may get distracted quite easily. So make sure to remove everything that may generate noise from the spot including your pet. Over a period of time, you can introduce some noise or activity so that he learns to focus even in the presence of distractions and thus the concentration becomes stronger.
- It is suggested that a child should start doing this for 3 to 5 minutes initially and then increase it to number of minutes that represent his age. For instance, if your child is 8, he should strong sit for 8 minutes and if he is 10, then it should be done for 10 minutes. However, it should be noted that the child should not strong sit beyond 20 minutes.
- While your child does strong sitting for reactive attachment disorder treatment, don't express any pessimism even if you notice something discouraging. At the same time, do not leave the child in complete control of his own. Act as a barely-there coach. For instance, if he doesn't want to strong sit, he may scratch his body or fidget. In this situation, you can indulge though make sure he resumes in 5 minutes. This is very important for if you succumb to his pressure every time he expresses reluctance to strong sit, he may take it as your weakness and look for excuse every time you tell him to do so.
- If your child is not able to do the entire thing, let him do weak sitting in the proportion of 3:1. It means he can either sit strong for 20 minutes or do weak sitting for one hour. In such a situation, he is

most likely to choose strong sitting. If he doesn't agree to finish his strong sitting, remind him politely that he needs to stay in his room and take rest until he becomes strong enough for this.

These are a few things which you need to take care of while the child is strong sitting for RAD treatment. These will surely help you in this task.

Attachment Therapists can help

Children do not develop symptoms of Reactive Attachment Disorder overnight. It is a gradual process, during which the affected child will start showing the symptoms slowly but steadily. There is no need of getting overwhelmed by the situation. What parents need to watch is, whether the behavioral disorders shown by your child have got any resemblance to the so called RAD symptoms. You will find a lot of websites that discuss about these symptoms in details. Go through them and find if the symptoms shown by your child are somewhat similar. If it is so, you should start looking for a competent Reactive Attachment Disorder therapist instead of taking a 'wait and watch' policy. Now the question here is how to look for a therapist who will be able to take care of your child and guide him or her out of this doldrums.

One of the best places to look for a Reactive Attachment Disorder therapist is the internet. You will find a number of them. Everyone will apparently appear to be expert enough to handle the situation but you must talk to them and find the one who has the most impressive credentials for the task. In most cases, it is seen that a general psychiatrist or psychologist is unable to carry out attachment therapy effectively and there have been cases, when they have misdiagnosed children over a prolonged period of time, contributing to the worsening of the situation.

- In case your child is showing the development of RAD symptoms, talk extensively to the therapists you find on the internet, fix an appointment with as many of them as possible, meet them in person and see if they are competent enough for treating your child. You can also refer to the feedbacks that are left by those who have enjoyed the service of the attachment therapist in past.
- Talking in person to the ones who have taken the service of a therapist will also help you immensely. These people will act as referrals largely due to the fact that these individuals were not trained to take care of children with symptoms of Reactive Attachment Disorder and they wholly depended on the therapists. They will provide you invaluable tips and information about how to find a competent Reactive Attachment Disorder therapist.
- If you cannot find any such suggestion from any quarter and your internet browsing session is of little help to you, you can call the Attachment center nearest to your address. They will make arrangements to put your child under treatment of a competent attachment therapist.
- You can also contact those who write articles and books on attachment therapy. They will definitely have the contact numbers of disorder therapists whom they train. Even if you find them staying miles apart, they might know a Reactive Attachment Disorder therapist who stays just a few blocks from your address.

Once you have found a therapist who is ready to take care of your child, there are a few things that you must do in advance, to make sure that your child is in safe hands. Let us discuss them in brief.

- Find out what the mentors the therapist has been trained under and research them thoroughly
- See if the Reactive Attachment Disorder therapist you have zeroed on is associated with Association for Treatment and Training in the Attachment of Children (ATTACh)
- Is the therapist working under the supervision of any senior therapist?
- Does the therapist have a degree or certificate from any workshop or a seminar specializing in RAD?
- Thoroughly go through the attachment therapy techniques that the therapist will follow and make sure that you agree with the techniques.

Last, but not the least, once you have found a competent Reactive Attachment Disorder therapist, don't expect results overnight. It is a long process. Keep in touch with the therapist and this will help you to keep track of the gradual improvement of your child. Disorder therapy is a continuous process and should not be expected to be over with within a few sessions.

RAD is caused by a Lack of Love and Affection

Right after birth, what a child needs the most is the tender touch of its mother, followed by other members of the family. As the child grows up, the care and affection provided by the family members helps him to develop of inter-personal bond. Thereafter, as the child grows up and establishes relations with the society, the interpersonal bond gets firmer. The platform of this entire concept is based on what the child faces during the first few years of its life. Understandably, any fallacy or defect or deprivation of love that the child receives during this initial period leaves a deep scar on the psychology, resulting in development of certain symptoms, namely that of Reactive Attachment Disorder develops.

This is the reason why the orphans or children of couples having a troubled marriage tend to develop symptoms of Reactive Attachment Disorder. Deprivation of love or a proper affection and tender physical touch from family members during the childhood days results in emotional poverty which sometimes takes turn to violent behavior when the child grows up. This is another very common symptom of Reactive Attachment Disorder. A thorough study on the orphans who are deprived of love and affection of parents have shown that these children are mentally crippled to develop any interpersonal bondage or respond and interact appropriately in any social gathering. They suffer from a crippling incapacity to create and maintain the normal emotional bondages that form the normal social existence of a human being.

On the other hand a child who is deprived of emotional and physical proximity during the days following birth tends to grow an extraordinary urge for affection that is coupled by a paradoxical phobia towards love and affection. It had a puzzling effect on the psyche and this is what the patients of Reactive Attachment Disorder generally show. As this urge to be loved and love does not fulfill when the individual grows up, that leads to extreme frustration in the subconscious mind along with a general precursor of anger, certain patients of Reactive Attachment Disorder get prone to periodical violent acts.

The less care that a child gets during the early days, the less they become capable of reciprocating it. Studies have revealed that the parents who were notorious enough to abuse their children physically and mentally were themselves seriously deprived of intimate physical affection and generally had poor sexual lives. So, in one sense they are themselves patients of Reactive Attachment Disorder. So it is perhaps not wrong to conclude that RAD and RAD symptoms are carried over from one generation to another till the chain is interrupted by someone with the help of proper diagnosis.

Hence, in order to get rid of the symptoms of Reactive Attachment Disorder, what is needed by a child is an affectionate environment in which the family members should leave no stones unturned to provide unconditioned love and affection to the new born and make sure that the mental development takes place in a proper way. Consulting a child psychologist during this stage is an imperative to be on the safer side.

Utilizing EMDR as RAD Treatment

One of the recently found treatments for RAD patients is EMDR. EMDR stands for "Eye Movement Desensitization and Reprocessing." It is a clinical treatment that has been devised to help children with reactive attachment disorder. This treatment can also be successfully used on the victims of sexual abuse, combat, domestic violence, and crime. In addition, individuals having addictions, depression, phobias, and low self-esteem issues can also be helped with this treatment. The importance of EMDR is being greatly realized nowadays. However, it should be noted that this treatment cannot be done at home.

EMDR is a complex and developed form of psychotherapy, in which other therapeutic methods involving eye movements or other types of rhythmical stimulation are combined to induce the ability of the brain to process information. All attachment therapists cannot offer this treatment of RAD. Only those who are trained or possess approval for providing EMDR therapy should be approached because this therapy cannot be given to all the patients with reactive attachment disorder.

As an effective treatment for trauma patients, the importance of EMDR is that it facilitates the eye movement of the patients in various directions as well as stimulates the brain bilaterally while the patient focuses on the disturbing things or materials. According to medical experts, traumatic moments get fixed or frozen in time. Some particular sounds, images, smells and feelings remind the patient, who is suffering from any traumatic experience in life, of the past moments that were not pleasant. These memories create a lasting impact on the mind of the person in a negative way and affect his perception about the world and other people who are a part of his or her life.

EMDR helps patients to get out of the depressing thoughts when those familiar sounds, images, smells or feelings are experienced yet again. The victim might encounter similar traumatic feelings but the impact is cut down considerably. Those who are recommended this therapy may have to attend 3 to 10 sessions. The sessions are conducted every week or on alternate weeks.

Furthermore, other than being a RAD treatment, EMDR can also treat several other medical conditions of the patients. These include:

- Depression
- Behavioral Issues
- Anxiety
- Death
- Discipline
- Trauma
- Verbal and Emotional Abuse
- Adoption Issues

Before going for this therapy, it's important that the patient asks himself a few questions and if the answer is 'yes' to any of the questions, then only EMDR should be considered as useful. The questions are:

- Is the practice of positive thinking not helpful enough for you to come out of depression and the feeling of loneliness?
- Do you want to know the main cause of chronic symptoms?
- Do you feel angry every time without knowing the reason behind it?
- Are the symptoms of anxiety affecting your life both at home and work?
- Are you not able to overcome your phobias even after putting your best efforts?
- Do you want to get rid of stress and its harmful impact on your physical health?

The importance of EMDR cannot be denied. However, before going for this therapy, you should ask yourself these and few other questions. When you feel confident enough to go to therapy, go ahead.

Caring for Children with RAD

Children, who are suffering from Reactive Attachment Disorder, need to have special care. That is quite obvious but it is also easier said than done. Statistics show that children suffering from RAD are generally very tough to handle. The reason behind this is that these kids are suspicious of virtually everything that goes on around them and are often found complaining about everything. They are not ready to share anything with anyone and are hesitant about developing any relationship whatsoever. Shouting at them or scolding is not advisable as this will only help them turn violent and make the matter worse.

First of all, you need a lot of patience and a fair amount of compassion while dealing with these children. More importantly, you need to use your brain to make that the kids suffering from Reactive Attachment Disorder feel at ease. For example, you can play a game with them, in order to make a difference. You can tell them to prepare a unique recipe no one has ever heard of! This may be quite interesting for them and will keep them enthralled. Tell them to take a piece of paper and write down the ingredients of the recipe. In this way, you can test their creative skills and keep them engaged in something innovative that will help them beat the symptoms of Reactive Attachment Disorder.

You can start of like this – tell them to use love, care and respect towards others, kisses for the loved ones, joy and happiness, honesty, forgiveness and fun, goodness and love and respect for God, healthiness and cleanliness, sympathy and empathy, a sense of responsibility and peace as ingredients! They will find this extremely interesting.

Once they have chalked down these 'ingredients', tell them to use their wit and intelligence to mix them up in the right amount and proportion to prepare the unique 'recipe' you are in search of. Once that is done, tell them that this recipe is not a food for stomach but a food for thought. That means the kids need to nurture it and memorize it properly so that they can utilize it in their lives to battle the ill effects of the ailment they are suffering from.

Routine treatment or counseling can be, at times, boring and too monotonous for the patients of Reactive Attachment Disorder who already have a propensity of getting impatient a bit too often. That is why innovative treatment and counseling concepts like the one described above can make a lot of difference so far as the result of the treatment is concerned. Moreover, because of its innovative and unique nature, this process will be able to draw a lot of attention from the patients of RAD, who seem to be living in a hopeless condition, having lost all the positive zeal to live life.

This is only an example of an innovative concept of treating Reactive Attachment Disorder. Similarly, you can surely invent your own ideas of treating these RAD affected kids to make sure that they can find a new way of starting off with their lives afresh!

RAD: In Adults

Reactive Attachment Disorder or RAD is a very serious and a somewhat rare mental disorientation generally found in children. The ailment crops up due to inability in forming normal inter-personal attachment with the ones who are generally associated during childhood. They include the immediate family members like mother, father, brother or sister. Experiences of negligence, abuse or violence or frequent change of care givers during early childhood days (especially between 6 months and 3 years) can lead to mental detachment or separation. This may ultimately result in problems in the communicative efforts of the child.

Though this ailment is generally associated with children, prolonged study has now revealed that adults fall victim to it as well. Problems that lead to Reactive Attachment Disorder are generally found to be in troublesome relationships on the professional and domestic fronts. It is also seen that adults who have suffered RAD during their childhood have shown reactive attachment disorder symptoms when they have grown up. The relationship patterns that these people have learned during their early childhood days continue to have a negative effect on them even during the later part of their lives. This becomes more evident during establishing relationship in their domestic & professional lives. At times, they pass these symptoms to their children, dragging the symptoms through generations till it is intervened and broken.

An adult who is suffering from Reactive Attachment Disorder can pose a serious threat to his or her children. This is because the individual is unable to establish a strong bondage and healthy relationship with them, causing the children to ultimately suffer from the same disorder. Since the first relationship that an infant gets into after birth, is with its parents, any problem in that relation affects the mental structure of the infant severely. This in turn has its effect at the time of the infant's upbringing. The child will refrain from growing any bondage with parents and other people the child comes in contact with.

It is seen that parents who are suffering from Reactive Attachment Disorder are generally hurtful and possess neglectful attitudes towards their children. They are abusive and at times even violent to their children though at times they are also seen to be clinging, co dependent and needy. All these prevent the child from getting close to their parents. Quite obviously, the children of these parents live life rather superficially. Being unable to have access and control of their emotions, they ultimately get isolated causing further deteriorating of their mental health.

Broadly, symptoms of reactive attachment disorder can be divided into two categories – Avoidant and Anxious or Ambivalent.

The Avoidant symptoms of Reactive Attachment Disorder include intense hostility and anger with a propensity of overt criticism of things and individuals and a tendency to blame others. Lack of sympathy and empathy, rendering others untrustworthy and undependable, loss of self-love and self-importance are also symptoms of

Avoidant Reactive Attachment Disorder. Besides, obsessive self-reliance, passive withdrawal from normal activities, avoiding intimacy in relationships, extreme difficulty in mingling and gelling with colleagues and co-workers are the other symptoms.

Some of the Anxious or Ambivalent symptoms include obsessive care towards a particular person, a sense of over-involvement or under-appreciation in relation, strong desire for a partner for relationship reciprocation. A strong desire for establishing excessive contact or declaration of love and affection, sensitivity to rejection, jealousy, overt possessiveness and show of extreme emotions are some other symptoms of Anxious or Ambivalent Reactive Attachment Disorder.

Professionals Writings about RAD

Our site has become one of the most trusted and viewed websites related to childhood disorders and various types of psychological disorders that people may encounter on a daily basis. Be it relatively complicated cases of Reactive Attachment Disorder or Attention Deficit Hyperactivity Disorder, or relatively common cases of Depression, this site has been playing the role of a perfect guide in helping people avail proper tips and suggestion about treating these ailments. Over a considerable period of time, the number of visitors to our site has increased to a considerable extent and a sizeable proportion of them are the friends or the family members of kids and adults suffering from one type of psychological disorder or the other.

Again, there are a few people who research our site who are not dealing with any cases of Nonverbal Learning Disorder, Asperger's Syndrome, or any other type of diseases, but are still eager to understand things about different psychological disorders. There are a few who are treating patients who have been erroneously diagnosed and would like to make amends and look for the right methods.

We regularly publish articles written by expert therapists and counselors for the benefit of our viewers. Therefore, we are appealing to the therapists and professionals with relevant experience of treating various types of articles with suggestions and tips of treatment so that we can serve our viewers in a much better way. We will be more than happy to publish them and accredit you for your articles.

How Strong Sitting can help Children with RAD

Strong Sitting is regarded as an extremely effective tool when it comes to treating children suffering from Reactive Attachment Disorder. It is a technique that is based on meditation and it helps kids with RAD in relaxing. It also helps the frontal portion of their brains to function properly. Research has revealed that when it comes to treating RAD in kids, strong sitting is an extremely handy technique that can make wonders. This technique assists the children suffering from RAD by controlling the flight behavior of their brain stem. Children who are suffering from Reactive Attachment Disorder generally live in an extremely chronic state of mind and anxiety coupled with a sense of fear and a hyper-vigilance. Doctors nowadays prescribe strong sitting to counter RAD as it helps these children to function normally brining the frontal part of the brain into normalcy in terms of functionality.

Strong sitting can be exercised in different times during the day as per the conveyance of the child in question. However, morning is the best time to exercise strong sitting. As everyone stays in a positive frame of mind at the start of the day, doing strong sitting during morning has an extremely positive effect on the mind, body and spirit of the affected child. Doctors say that kids with RAD should religiously exercise strong sitting to counter RAD at the mornings to optimize its effects. They should do it after they get up from the bed or after they have come back from the bathroom.

Strong sitting can also be done after a session of acting out. After acting out episode, carrying out strong sitting can bring back the frontal lobe of the brain into normalcy bringing some amount of sanity in the child.

Whenever that is done, make sure that your child develops a regular habit of strong sitting. At first, kids with RAD should sit for a minute and then after the kid gets habituated with it, the time should be increased gradually. Things are easier said than done. To begin with, the child might be distracted quite easily but with time, as the habits grow stronger the kid becomes calmer and mentally stronger to ignore such distractions.

Again, you need to be as creative as possible. As your kid gets mentally used to sitting, you may introduce certain distractions during the sitting. Make sure that the distractions are as natural and as obvious as the ones you encounter in your daily lives and see how your child reacts. The idea is to make your child suffering from Reactive Attachment Disorder to focus as much as possible during the sitting as things go on taking place around him or her as usual. This will make your kid stronger and gain more concentration and remain calm.

You should take note that the strong sitting is done in a correct manner with correct posture. See if the child is cool, calm and still, relaxed with a normal belly breathing to optimize the results. Strong sitting will do wonders for arresting the symptoms of Reactive Attachment Disorder in children.

Craniosacral Therapy

Whether craniosacral therapy is effective or not is little controversial issue, but its usefulness in treating RAD patients cannot be denied. In fact, this therapy is found effective in case of several other medical conditions also relating to dysfunction and pain. Through this gentle and hands-on therapy, the function of the craniosacral system including membranes and cerebrospinal fluid that cover and shield the brain and spinal cord is evaluated and improved.

In this method, practitioners use soft and gentle touch to let go of restrictions in the craniosacral system and ensure enhancement of the central nervous system. Craniosacral therapy can be learnt at home. However, it's important that the person who teaches you this technique is well qualified and has some hands-on experience in this field. The person from whom you learn this technique can be an attachment therapist for children. Though there are many people who think that the basis of this therapy is false, it's getting popular nowadays and is believed to cause no harm if done properly.

On the basis of personal experiences, some people have the opinion that this therapy is useful for patients who have undergone RAD diagnosis. It creates an opportunity for physical closeness and can open up a way for attachment for these patients. In RAD treatment, this therapy plays a useful function by giving a child an opportunity to get close to someone in a peaceful environment.

Now, the question is – who can take advantage from craniosacral therapy? According to some medical experts, this therapy is meant for everyone including reactive attachment disorder patients. The results this therapy produces can bring dramatic changes in the patients suffering from dryness, memory loss, aging, violence, accidents, birth trauma, etc. The good thing about this therapy is that it builds up the brain and nervous system of the patient and creates a secure environment in which the patient's body can exhibit the unresolved issues and the practitioner can find out a resolution.

Benefits of Craniosacral Therapy

There are many benefits attached to this therapy. The craniosacral therapists say that this treatment can prove effective in relieving pain, chronic fatigue, hyperactivity, depression, and several other medical conditions which can be damaging for immune, nervous or endocrine systems. But since the craniosacral model is quite different from the scientific medical framework, the results cannot be determined by scientific trials.

The benefits of craniosacral therapy are a contentious issue with both scientific researchers and medical experts because it doesn't conform to the health model used in western medical science. Nevertheless, there are few studies which acknowledge its effectiveness in relieving chronic pain and curing trauma and stress related disorders. Since there is no single opinion about the effectiveness of this model, it is better that you consult your primary health care physician before undergoing this therapy for alleviating a health condition. The physician can tell you whether this therapy will be right for your medical condition and can also refer you to a proper medical center.

Tips on how to handle RAD

Reactive Attachment Disorder is a rather uncommon mental disorder that begins to affect children from an early age onward; there are a variety of reasons in which a child is affected by this. Hence, when it comes to tackling RAD, affected the parents of affected children should follow certain techniques in order to make sure the ailment is keep under control.

- First of all, they need to be optimistic and look for a positive outcome, even if the result is temporary.
- Think about innovative ideas that will get the child in question into a comfort zone. This is the most important thing to help the kid feel at ease and mentally comfortable. As Reactive Attachment Disorder is an absolutely psychological ailment, the mental state of the child will always make a difference.
- They can also join forums of other parents who are tackling RAD. They can join the discussion and can be aware of various innovative concepts of tackling Reactive Attachment Disorder.

- One of the most important things that the parents should keep in mind while handling Reactive Attachment Disorder is having realistic expectations. They should not expect overnight results. Guiding the Reactive Attachment Disorder affected kids is a long and continuous process and they should not lose focus during the long course to taste success at the end of the road.
- One the same note, patience is something that is the key of treating Reactive Attachment Disorder. As the entire process of tackling RAD is time consuming, the parents will have to show immense patience before the techniques adopted will start yielding any results.
- Keeping the kid in question in a jovial mood is another very important aspect of treatment. Hence, it is absolutely imperative that an atmosphere of joy and humor is maintained in the house and when dealing with the kid. This will help in the treatment in a long way and repair the problems of mental attachment that the kid might have with the other members of the family. It is also needed to have at least two to three people always in jovial mood around the kid affected by Reactive Attachment Disorder.
- It is important for the parents not get bogged down or lose hearts. They should take care of themselves to reduce the mental stress that the entire situation might have caused. A good amount of rest along with timely intake of healthy and nutritious meals, and relaxation are also as important as tackling RAD. It is important to recharge their batteries before tackling Reactive Attachment Disorder.
- It is also important to seek help from outside – mainly from friends, relatives, various community

resources. This is needed to avoid excessive mental stress while treating Reactive Attachment Disorder.
- Staying positive and never losing hope is another key to success in tackling RAD. Losing hope will not make the situation better and only put the child into further doldrums. At the same time, being sensitive to the child's feelings is also needed. It will only encourage the child and provide the required assurance that is the need of the hour for the kid.

Dealing with RAD patients who steal

It will be difficult to be a parent of a RAC child; there are many reasons that this may be difficult. Children with RAD symptoms tend to be emotionally unattached with their parents and caregivers, they can misbehave with them, they resist any kind of love and affection coming from them, etc. At certain point of time, such behaviors start taking a toll even on the relationships of their parents with others in the family, leading to frustration and the feeling of helplessness. However, if the RAD child has the habit of stealing, then the task becomes all the more challenging for parents. In such a situation, anyone can lose control or feel defeated. But, if you want you can help your child to end his stealing tendency. For this, you would have to keep certain things in mind. To help you a bit, some points are discussed below.

Why do some RAD children develop tendencies of stealing?

A child who is diagnosed with the symptoms of RAD tends to steal things to alleviate their internal stress level and mood swings. When he picks a thing which is not his own, he experiences a powerful chemical reaction within. The degree of reaction can differ from individual to individual. The more he indulges in this, the more he develops an addiction for it. His system starts responding to such behavior. He feels an internal urge to put the object in this pocket so that everything goes okay, if not more than at least for 5 minutes. When emotional deregulation again takes place in him, he may again go for stealing things.

A child may also steal as a reaction to certain events, environments or situations. For instance, some children find it easy to steal from stores and other, from teacher's desk due to overwhelming stimulation or conditioning. The reason behind this can be stress. A child may find it stressful to be in such a particular kind of environment and hence, to ease himself, he starts stealing.

When any such symptoms are noticed in reactive attachment disorder children, parents need to take concrete and constructive steps to help their little ones come out of this.

How can one deal with RAD children who steal?

While dealing with such tendencies in a RAD child, it's important that you maintain your cool and stay calm. Don't blame your child, instead talk to him. Tell him that "he puts things which are not his in his pockets when he is stressed out. By doing this, you feel good. But this can hurt others. When you are scared or stressed out, come to me." You have to make him understand this and also tell him that next time when he goes to a store, you will be with him by his side. Similarly, if teachers are aware of the mental condition of your child, they can also help him with their affection and understanding. Hugging and talking instead of punishing the child can lead to positive results.

Another step that can be taken towards dealing with reactive attachment disorder children is that of building the level of tolerance in them. For example, first time when you accompany him to a store where he doesn't feel comfortable, make sure to hold his hands. It will be comforting. Next time simply stand with him and gradually increase your distance little by little. While practicing this step, be patient and calm.

Attachment Therapy for RAD children

The evolution of attachment therapy cannot be denied. With constant revision, research and evaluation, medical experts have developed such methodologies in this therapy which facilitate the process of treating RAD patients. However, due to continuous changes in the methodology, some people find it difficult to accept its importance and efficacy in healing severe medical conditions. In fact, it has become a much debated issue in paramedical system among a number of people including those parents who are coping up with their RAD children.

It is necessary to point out that changes in the methodology cannot be considered as wrong because discovering the best ways to reach out to the children with reactive attachment disorder is most important. Some experts believe that the main cause of confusion about this therapy can be partly attributed to misinformation and misinterpretation. To be precise, let's consider the case of "holding therapy". This technique in attachment therapy is meant to foster the bond between a mother and her child. In this therapy, the mother holds her child in a nurturing position. The process includes smiles, voice, touch, eye contact and movement, recreating the feeling of safety and security in the mind of the child, transporting back in time when this bonding should have happened.

Another attachment therapy that is used much like the "holding therapy" in the treatment of RAD patients is called "rebirthing". In this technique, a womb-like environment is recreated to help child feel his birth experience and attach to his primary caregivers. Alas, this therapy is supposed to have caused at least two deaths of the children, one in Utah and another in Colorado, from suffocation due to the use of blanket which is needed to stimulate the womb. But for these deaths, the use of this therapy cannot be disparaged. The main reason was the involvement of an unlicensed therapist in one case and in another case it was a parent who tried to conduct this procedure in the absence of a child's therapist. Anyway, the rebirthing method is not used anymore in larger potions due to these deaths and continuing controversy.

There is one more attachment therapy called "re-parenting". Most people confuse this technique of RAD treatment with rebirthing, despite the fact that re-parenting is not at all life-threatening. Through this therapy, the child with attachment disorder is helped to experience the primary cares of early life which are vital for attachment. These include rocking in the lap, holding, feeding from a feeding bottle and signing rhymes by a parent. Other than this, parents are also asked to play games with him like hide-and-seek and reading stories at night. All the things that a RAD child could not experience in his early life are done to help him attach with the caregivers.

Parenting a RAD child is not easy and hence, it is understandable that any parent would like to try things that promise to make their child's life healthy and comfortable. But it's important to note that before making any decision, you should always consult your child's therapist so that he/she can suggest the most suitable attachment therapy for him and at the same time, guide you on the changes that need to be implemented in your parenting style.

Breaking down the barriers between you and your RAD child

A reactive attachment disorder child will try very hard to push you away from himself. However, for the well-being of the child, you need to make stronger efforts in order to ensure the removal of attachment barriers between you and your child.

You cannot win his love by offering him privileges or things. It will anyway not ensure good behavior, healing or attachment. In fact, the privileges and things which you buy for him may later stand in the way of your relationship with him. And then, this may only reinforce negative behavior in child and hamper the process of healing. Instead, wait for the right time.

You need to keep this in mind that your relationship with your kid and his healing is the priority. You need to consider the misbehavior of your child as learning experience for yourself without getting hurt. Don't allow anger to impede the progress of healing.

Electronic Devices: Television, Video Games, Computers, and Radios

These electronic devices can only create barriers in the way of relationships, thought and emotions even of a healthy child. If you are bringing up a RAD child, make sure to remove various barriers of attachment which include these electronic devices. Either keep them somewhere or don't allow your child to use it much. Remove these distractions until your child is back to normalcy and the mutual relationship between you and him is strong.

If your child is healthy, the use of these devices, such as, video games and television should be restricted to two hours per week. As far as the RAD child is concerned, he should not be allowed to watch television for 6 months to 1 year. He and his brain should be given an opportunity to develop the ability to process information. It will facilitate his healing process as well.

If the complete removal of attachment barriers such as, television or radio is not possible, then, restrict the amount of time he spends with these and keep a watch over the kind of programs he watches. Cartoons with faster flicker rates are not good for him.

Instead of permitting your child to spend time with electronic devices, encourage him to play with problem-solving toys, such as, Legos, Lincoln Logs, and Constructs, etc.

Furniture and Other Household Items

Children with attachment disorders tend to destroy things. Hence, while trying to improve their behavior, consider replacing expensive products with less expensive ones that may include even secondhand unbreakable furniture. This is required to be done especially in the child's room. Usually, it's better to not clutter his room much. Expect the child to get rid of anything that he can vandalize or demolish, but don't let your relationship with your child get affected in your effort to save your furniture.

Friends and Close Ones

The relationship between your child and his friends can again be one of the RAD attachment barriers for you. The emotional connect between you and your child would diminish further if you allow him to speak with his friends over phone or go outside with them. Since a RAD child has the potential to be charming, he will like to be friends with those kids who are not emotionally demanding. The more he will mingle with them, the more he will get convinced that you are over demanding of him.

Another issue is that older adolescent and teens can be good at flirting. And if they start getting responses, the emotional gap at home may get further open up. Therefore, you need to ensure that you don't give your child any unwarranted privileges. Restrict the time he spends with his friends alone or over the phone. In fact, you can ask his friends to visit your house and spend some time with your child under your vigilance, rather than allowing your kid to go out with them. This will help you monitor him. Also, don't let your child avoid family outings for movies, restaurant or church.

Games

Instead of letting your child play games alone, encourage him to spend time playing games which need participation from two or more members of the family. This will be very useful for all of you. So as a part of attachment barrier removal tactics, you can keep cribbage, Monopoly and other popular games in and around your house. Make sure that your child participates in the game with full enthusiasm. To ensure the removal of attachment barriers while playing games with him, you can use conversation and strategy sharing as a powerful weapon.

Writings on RAD

Children who suffer from Reactive Attachment Disorder at times behave rather erratically, shouting at things, and at times making moves that may sometimes appear to be extremely insulting and embarrassing for anyone. However, these spells do not last forever and soon the kids calm down. Once the temper cools off, these kids with RAD even feel sorry for their behavior. However, in most of the times, they find it difficult to express themselves and their thoughts while apologizing for what they have done.

Taking this into consideration, experts believe that the best thing that these kids with Reactive Attachment Disorder can be told to do is to write down their feelings. This will have a two pronged effect on the kids. Firstly, they will be able to utilize their thoughts in a coordinated way to create something innovative and secondly and most importantly, they will be able to express themselves in a much better way which should make them feel better.

A prolonged research has revealed that when children suffer from RAD write down these kinds of stuffs, only 5 per cent of the entire contents are serious stuffs while the rest is found to be fillers and expression of some distorted thought processes. All said and done, these writings help the therapists and counselors a lot in gauging the mental state of the Reactive Attachment Disorder patients. Naturally, diagnosis becomes much easier.

On our website, you will find articles written by experts on RAD. We sincerely hope that these articles will help people get a lot of information and tips regarding tackling children suffering from Reactive Attachment Disorder. R.D. Laing is one of them, whose articles are extremely valuable when it comes to guiding parents of kids who are suffering from RAD.

We, hereby, welcome parents and people tackling cases of Reactive Attachment Disorder to share more of their experiences along with essays written by their kids suffering from RAD so that people going through our website can get a firsthand experience of what goes on across the mind of an affected child. This will help them to coup with the situation much better.

Identify RAD symptoms

The main cause of reactive attachment disorder (RAD) in children can be attributed to the experience of trauma in life. The impact of this disorder can be mild as well as severe depending on the extent and duration of the experience of trauma. Usually, medical health experts associate abandonment as the root cause of this psychological condition in children. Other than this, abuse and neglect at a very early stage of life can also be held responsible for the occurrence of such ailment. RAD symptoms can become worse if a child's traumatic experiences are not tackled in time, especially in case the ailment has been caused by experience(s) that the victim has met with at early stages of life.

The best way to detect the symptoms of reactive attachment disorder in a child is through diagnosis. During diagnosis, assessing the child's history and the current symptoms the victim is showing is important. Medical health experts believe that diagnosis should be based on the information provided by the child's parents, instead of the perception of the clinician. The reason being, children with RAD can fake or manipulate their behavior to appear good.

There are some other ways which can help you to identify the signs and symptoms of RAD during early childhood.

Signs and Symptoms

A child with RAD conditions faces developmental difficulty in social interactions and the signs start showing even before he turns 5. The indication of this is your kid's constant failure to respond appropriately to the normal social interactions that a child should do at that age. The kid can be hyper vigilant, extremely ambivalent, as well as, inhibited. The responses can well be contradictory. This becomes clear when a child tries to avoid any kind of love and comfort coming from the caregivers, exhibits frozen behavior, and remains unattached to other members of the family. Besides, a RAD child may find difficulty in selecting attachment figures. For instance, the child may get over attached to strangers while feeling no attachment towards family members or the ones whom the kid knows.

However, developmental delays alone cannot be taken as the sole indication of reactive attachment disorder in a child. Other factors also need to be evaluated as well. For instance, a child can develop such mental condition if the expectations in terms of affection, comfort and nurturing are not met. Not getting enough care from the primary caregivers or frequent changes in foster care system can also lead to this kind of mental health condition.

If you find all of these symptoms in your child, then, it's probably time that you should take him or her to see professional medical help. The symptoms of reactive attachment disorder can be arrested with appropriate treatment. Usually, in this treatment, involvement of both patients and their families is what is most required. A medical health expert can recommend several types of psychotherapy, trainings and counseling for your child.

Diagnosis also includes training and counseling classes for both the patients and their parents and other members of the family. The treatment may include family therapy, individual psychological counseling, parenting skills classes, and so on. These methods of treatment are basically adopted to help a RAD child improve the relationship with the peer groups and to enhance self-esteem.

RAD Cool down Techniques

Reactive attachment disorder (RAD) is a mental health condition in which infants or young children find themselves unable to establish any relationship with parents or adults. This condition can be found to develop in children who were abused or neglected during early childhood and have spent their lives in foster care. Similarly, children from orphanages can also be seen to have this kind of mental ailment. According to medical experts, the condition of RAD develops when children's basic needs for comfort, affection and nurturing are not satisfied. As a result of this, these children fail to establish any bondage with their parents or caregivers and their brain development also gets affected. It's a permanent condition, but with proper treatment the child can be taught to build healthy and stable relationships both at home and school. For treating reactive attachment disorder child, parent training, school training and psychological counseling are required.

A child who is suffering from this disorder may face difficulty in controlling his anger, physical habits, talking, cravings, etc. In order to help the child, you need to teach him certain techniques of discipline at home, public places and school. Your child will get the taste of success once he is aware of the tools which he can use to evaluate every situation and control his actions to cope up with the resulting impulses. One of such techniques is RAD cool down ideas.

Cool down Ideas for a Child who has RAD

If your child is unable to react calmly to heated situations, teach him the techniques to cool down rather than responding in an improper way. Assign your child a particular place in the house and send the child there whenever he's arguing with any member of the family. Equip him with self-control techniques such as deep breathing exercises while looking at a particular object in distance or doing backward counting from 100. This will help him calm down in public places as well as at home. While providing this RAD treatment, you can ask your child to follow the below mentioned steps.

RAD Cool down Techniques

- *Ask your child to do deep breathing thrice.*
- *Ask him to follow this list*:
  - I am feeling mad and these feelings are okay.
  - Tell the adults that I need some time to think before I talk. Most adults even do the same.
  - After I calm down, I feel happy and proud of myself and I did not disregard myself or other family members when I was angry.
  - If I disrespected someone, sit for a longer period of time and repeat it to myself that I made a mistake,

but keep in mind that mistakes can be corrected by imbibing the right behavior.
- ✓ Note down the kind of right behavior I should have followed when I was feeling angry and practice it in future when I have any such feeling.
- ✓ I should start doing the required thing when I calm down and feel respectful towards others.
- ✓ Sit a bit more if I don't calm down and feel respectful while thinking about a better time to get back at the thing that needs to be done. It's fine to spend quiet time in my room, just thinking.
- ✓ It's fine to say that I am feeling tired and I want to take rest or sleep. Let others know what my plans are.
- ➢ *Jot down in a diary or journal*:
- ✓ I wish…..
- ✓ I don't like it when….
- ✓ I am feeling mad because….
- ✓ I am happy or proud of myself because I did not disrespect or….
- ✓ These are the things which I think I can do next time ………

These are some of the RAD cool down steps, which, if followed by the child, can yield to desirable results.

Understanding how Eye Contact affects RAD Children

A reactive attachment disorder child finds it difficult to make proper eye contact while taking with adults. However, it is interesting to note that he might be successful in maintaining eye contact while interacting with his peers or strangers. He will make brilliant eye contact with you only when he is lying to you about something or trying to manipulate you.

Eye contact, which is often considered a strong tool in any situation, should always be demanded from children with RAD symptoms. The reason behind this is that eyes are considered to be the gateway to the soul. It's not only about looking at the child. It is all about looking with loving, strong and lively eyes to convey to him that everything is okay and he is safe. Repeating this time and again will help you reach the heart of your child and get through the mental barrier that he has created around him. Do this till he gets completely healed.

People using eye contact to treat RAD patients are aware that it's both a great expression of love as well as weapon. However, be careful while using your eyes to express something. An angry eye contact can damage your relationship with him rather than doing anything good. It is important to remember that the child with this kind of disorder does this in order to push you away.

You can demand your child to make eye contact with you while you both are talking to each other. Initially, the child may face certain difficulty in making eye contact, but insist on practicing this.

Also, do not allow your child to call you from another room when he desires to talk to you about something. Let him come to you and speak with a direct eye contact. If he faces any difficulty in doing this, help him practice. Send him to his living room and ask him to wait for your call. When he goes away, call him gently. If he responds, allow him to communicate with you while maintaining an eye contact. This should be practiced till the time he performs it correctly. While practicing this, make sure to use good amount of enthusiasm and positive support.

There is one more thing that you need to know about reactive attachment disorder eye contact. While your child communicates with you, insist that he has an eye contact with you. Don't acknowledge if he does otherwise. Look at his eyes with a smile in your eyes and don't allow yourself to get distracted by anything when you two are speaking.

It might not always be possible to make an eye contact every time he communicates, but try to implement this. A RAD child feels safe whenever an adult holds an authoritative position compared to any normal child who would prefer his parents to kneel down at their level.

You should not insist on making eye contact when he is frustrated or angry. At the same time, you should not expect your child to look into your eyes when you lose control because this would simply spoil all the efforts that you have made so far.

Nonverbal Learning Disorders

How to Help Children with Nonverbal Learning Disorders

Nonverbal Learning Disorders are one of the most frequent mental disorders that children tend to suffer from, especially, during their earliest years. It is quite obvious, that Nonverbal Learning Disorder treatment becomes imperative for these children. However, how a NLD affected child is being treated by their parents and other family members at home is also equally important, when it comes to evaluating the chances of recovery. Parents of a kid with Nonverbal learning disorder symptoms need to follow certain techniques when bringing up their kids. In fact, as per the experts, following the proper procedure of bringing these kids up is itself a part of Nonverbal learning disorder treatment.

The following are some of the aspects that a parent of a child who is suffering from a Nonverbal Learning Disorder should understand.

Putting maximum emphasis on the assets of the child

The first and foremost condition of upbringing a child with Nonverbal Learning Disorder is nurturing their strong areas properly. In other words, when you know that the disease may hinder certain types of activities of the child, or put his or her abilities in question, refrain the child from doing those activities – at least in the early stages of treatment. Instead, put increased focus on the stronger points that the kid might have and to nurture them. This will provide a lot of confidence and impart a sense of self-esteem in the child. At the same time, distract the child from the weaknesses and help him ignore them.

Show as much affection as possible

Never ever be harsh to the child who is suffering from Nonverbal Learning Disorder. This is the first and foremost condition of treating Nonverbal learning disorder. Be as much affectionate, loving and caring to your child as possible. The child may show marked difference from others, but that should not deter you from loving your child, especially if you have another kid who is normal. Give extra care to him or her whenever the need arises.

Impart a sense of independence while maintaining a strict vigil

What a kid with Nonverbal learning disorder symptoms needs is self confidence and self belief. That is why a constant attention and offer of help may have a negative impact on the child. This will stop self confidence from growing and this will harm the child in the long run. Therefore, while you continue to keep a watch on your child, importance should be given to see that he or she does everything independently, with least help from others. This will only increase the self confidence in the Nonverbal learning disorder patient.

Development of social skills:

This is another very important aspect of bringing up a kid with Nonverbal learning disorder symptoms. There is an ardent need of encouraging the kid to socialize and interact with people around him or her. Encouraging the child to develop relation with likeminded people or kids is the best way to develop the social skills.

The Impact of a NLD

When we discuss Nonverbal Learning Disorders, the first and foremost thing that comes into is its impact on the patient and a thorough analysis of these effects is necessary to better understanding these problems. The effects can be broadly differentiated into the following categories or criteria.

Criteria #1 –

A phenomenon that is fairly statistically uncommon

- This phenomenon clearly underlines the disparity between different intellectual or academic proficiency within the brain of the patient.
- Ability of the patient to perform various tasks that are related to linguistics in a much better way than the tasks which are not related to linguistics.

Criteria #2:

Impact of Nonverbal Learning Disorder on various activities

Mathematics –

While practicing mathematics, the patients would often be able to score high marks, especially during the early grades though they are often found wanting during the higher grades. The root cause of this problem is the nonverbal learning disability that affects the concepts of mathematics. They face hardship in understanding the calculations and related concepts. Instead, they develop a tendency of following a stereotype step-by-step methodology that is not always correct and that affects their performance.

Handwriting –

Patients of Nonverbal Learning Disorder, at times, find it difficult to start writing papers. This is more evident when they sit for a test. The patient would often find problem in automating functionalities of letters and alphabets. Organizing words and letters to form sentences also becomes extremely difficult for the patient. This is the most apparent symptom that the doctors look for at the time of Non Verbal Learning Disorder treatment.

Organization –

Children who are suffering from NLD generally face a lot of trouble in seeing through big tasks, especially, when these tasks constitute several smaller tasks. Cleaning a room as a whole, for instance might be quite a problematic task for them, though they would hardly find any problem in picking up and arranging things that are scattered all over the room. Another very familiar symptom of Nonverbal Learning Disorder is forgetting the ultimate bigger task on hand while concentrating on the smaller ones.

Attention –

Certain children, who are suffering from a nonverbal learning disability, face issues with paying attention.

However, they are mainly found to show this symptom only in those situations which are either too difficult for them to coup with or are too boring.

Socialization –

Thorough research on children, who are suffering from a nonverbal learning disability, has revealed that they are good when it comes to socializing, especially, during their early years. However, as they grow up and the complexity of their surroundings keeps on growing larger around them, they will find it increasingly difficult to keep up with. In particular, they often face immense problems in gauging and responding to non–verbal communicative gestures such as, various facial expressions, body language, voice intonations, choice of vocabulary, expression of eyes, picking up certain delicate tones such as, sarcasm and so on. This often lands them in utterly embarrassing situations which further affects their mindset.

Other factors that fall in this criterion are anxiety and fear, the lack of understanding non-verbal thought processes, and the lack of motor coordination.

Criteria #3:

The Absence of Alternative Explanations

The patients who have Nonverbal learning Disorders, suffer from this aberration, which results in intellectual disabilities, needless anxiety, inabilities to learn, or grasp the right opportunity to learn. Prolonged research has also revealed that Nonverbal Learning Disorder causes a Semantic-Pragmatic Language Disorder in children.

Because of this, the patients are unable to form complex languages. This leads to various types of problems in comprehension & socialization.

Criteria # 4:

A Steady Pattern of Developmental Disorders

Children suffering from Nonverbal Learning Disorders, at times, will show a consistent pattern of developmental aberration over a prolonged period of time.

ADHD

ADHD Causes

The frantic pace of modern life takes its toll on people, especially children who find it increasingly difficult to keep up. This, along with some other issues, results in the development of a variety of mental aberrations, of which Attention Deficit Hyperactivity Disorder or ADHD is one. The following are the primary causes of Attention Deficit Hyperactivity Disorder in children.

- *Diet*:
  One school of thought, which was propagated way back in the 70s, shares that one of the causes of Attention Deficit Hyperactivity Disorder is hypersensitivity of babies to certain ingredients of baby food that are consumed during their infant years. It also states that consumption of foods that are rich in sugar lead to certain impulsive & hyperactive behavior or children although no concrete proof has been found thereof. As such, this theory mainly remains a myth and was mainly fanned by the media rather than the experienced therapists and researchers.

- *Imbalance in hormonal secretion*:

  Mood swings and behavioral patterns of individuals are mainly governed by secretion of various types of hormones. Though there are contradicting theories of hormonal imbalance being one of the major ADHD causes this has not been proved yet. In fact, though hormonal imbalance is often held responsible for fickle mindedness or lack of focus and impulsive behavior, especially during puberty and adolescence, it is not found to have affected the symptoms of ADHD or the disorder itself.

- *Balance or Vestibular Problems*:
  The mental balance of an individual is chiefly controlled by the vestibular system of the brain. Hence, any aberration in that system should ideally kick off problems in behavior. From this concept, the researchers arrived at the theory that said Attention Deficit Hyperactivity Disorder is a type of motion sickness that is triggered off by a defect in the vestibular system. However, advanced research has dismissed this theory recently stating that there is no relation whatsoever between Attention Deficit Hyperactivity Disorder and the vestibular system of the brain.

- *Pattern of Family Life and Parenting*:
  This, according to modern researchers, is probably the main factor which causes Attention Deficit Hyperactivity Disorder. Improper ways of bringing up children, especially, by step mothers and step fathers is often the cause of Attention Deficit Hyperactivity Disorder. Again, a troubled marriage with rifts between the parents that extend up to separation can have adverse effects on the child, resulting in subsequent development of symptoms of ADHD. Adverse behavior by schoolmates or teachers, coupled with negligence

and lack of empathy in home, can also result in ADHD.

- *Watching too much TV*:

This is one of the most popular ADHD causes. Watching too much TV may cause children to be alienated from the family or social life, giving rise to symptoms of ADHD. Watching too much violence in TV can impart a sense of aggression in the child though, technically speaking, that cannot be termed as classical ADHD, though there are some similarities between the symptoms of hyperactivity and impulsiveness, which are exhibited by ADHD patients.

Importation Information in Understanding ADHD

Attention Deficit Hyperactivity Disorder (ADHD) is a severe medical condition which is found in many children and often, continues into adulthood. An ADHD patient finds difficulty in focusing on things and exhibits impulsion and hyperactive behaviors. Children who are diagnosed with this mental disorder can also face poor self-esteem, weak performance in school and relationship issues.

The main causes of attention deficit hyperactivity disorder can be attributed to heredity, certain structure of the brain, food additives, exposure to toxins, consumption of drugs, etc. The symptoms which can result from one or the combination of the aforementioned ADHD causes include inattentiveness, inability to perform tasks, a tendency to avoid tasks that need intense focus, distraction, forgetfulness, fidgeting, excessive talking, impatience, and poor social skills, etc.

This type of mental disease cannot be cured completely; however, there are some methods of treatment which can help patients. The main treatment includes medications and counseling. In addition, family and community support as well as special changes in the classroom can also work as a treatment for ADHD children.

In order to treat the symptoms of ADHD, a patient can be prescribed stimulant drugs or nonstimulant medication. The stimulant drugs may include Dextroamphetamine-amphetamine, Methylphenidate and Dextroamphetamine. These stimulants increase and regulate the percentage of brain chemicals known as neurotransmitters. With the help of these medicines, the signs and causes of impulsive and hyperactive behavior and inattention are treated. These medications can be effective for only a short period of time. Also, the doses are prescribed on a case-by-case basis. However, it's important to note that these medications can cause some side-effects and these include weight loss, poor or weak appetite, and irritability.

When stimulant medications don't work, then, ADHD patients are prescribed nonstimulant medications. In nonstimulant medications, Atomoxetine is usually applied. Besides reducing the severity of the ADHD symptoms, Atomoxetine reduces anxiety as well. If this medicine is taken once or twice a day, it can cause side effects like sedation, nausea, weight loss, decreased or poor appetite, etc. In addition to these, children with attention deficit hyperactivity disorder can also be given antidepressants, clonidine and guanfacine.

There are certain things that need to be taken care of in case of these medications. These are – the medicines should be kept in a childproof container, these should not be sent to school with the children and the doses should be carefully administered, strictly as per the prescription.

Apart from medication, children with attention deficit hyperactivity disorder can also be recommended behavior counseling or therapies. Some of these therapies are – psychotherapy, social skills training, parenting skills training, behavior therapy, support groups and family therapy.

If the issue of attention deficit hyperactivity disorder in children is addressed and taken care of by a team that consists of the parents, teachers, and therapists, the results can be expected to be good. Another thing which is important for proper treatment is that the condition of the patient should be thoroughly diagnosed. If diagnosis is accurate, the patient can be recommended medications and therapies which are most suitable for him. All these steps are crucial for ensuring a healthy lifestyle for ADHD patients.

Oppositional Deficient Disorder

Understanding the Differences between ODD and Normal Childhood Disobedience

From the ages of 6 to 12, many children will become disobedient. This is the period of their mental growth, in which they love to play pranks and be mischievous. However, this is also the age group when they tend to develop Oppositional Defiant Disorder symptoms. Hence, the million dollar question arises - how can you know if your child is just one of the naughty kids who love playing pranks on other or if they are victims of Oppositional Defiant Disorder.

Experts believe that simple disobedience has a lot of reasons behind it. One reason may be that the child may not have the willingness of being dominated by the parents and want to do something of his or her own. This may lead that child into doing something that the parents may not like. If that happens, that is just a case of disobedience and there is nothing to be worried about that. However, the ones with Oppositional Defiant Disorder are quite different. They develop a knack of constantly downplaying the authority of the parents and they develop a tendency that clearly says the parents are no more in charge of the proceedings. Now, this is quite alarming if it happens continuously. In fact, this is one of the primary symptoms of ODD.

Simple cases of depression will never be accompanied by depression and violence. However, kids with ODD symptoms have a tendency of growing deep emotional hurts. They tend to yearn for attention from everyone around them with a sense of fretfulness along with depression that is manifested by the conduct of the individual, every now and then. They feel that they are being neglected and hence, show a lot of violence at times. They envy their siblings and consider them as their rivals and often inflict harm upon them. At times Oppositional Defiant Disorder in extreme cases may be accompanied with Dyslexia and hearing impairment.

Children with Oppositional Defiant Disorder symptoms may also have problems in expressing their thoughts and emotions and that will never happen in cases of simple disobedience. As such, parents of these kids face a lot of challenge in bringing back the kid in question to normalcy. In these cases, early detection plays a pivotal role in helping the kid out of the wood. Early detection and quick action with the help of an experienced psychotherapist will help these kids in a tremendous way to come out of the effects of this dreadful ailment before it leaves any permanent scar on the mindset of the child.

However, in this, the parents will need to make sure that they are proactive. Care should be taken to ensure that the kids with ODD symptoms are never ill behaved with and more emphasis in given on the symptoms rather than the child. Constant communication should be maintained with the child to make sure the mental connection is never lost. Unconditional love and constant attention should be given so that the child never feels that he or she is of any less importance than the other members of the family.

Symptoms of ODD

Oppositional Defiant Disorder (ODD) is an enduring pattern of disobedience guided by anger and a viciously defiant behavior toward authority figures. These bouts of hostility at times cross the limits of the normal behavioral patterns of childhood. Children showing symptoms of ODD are generally extremely stubborn with an excessively violent attitude and temper. Let us discuss some of the symptoms of Oppositional Defiant Disorder that are commonly diagnosed.

Studies have revealed that children of couples who are having problematic relations or those of alcoholic parents generally have about 18% propensity of developing symptoms of ODD, at a very early age.

- The most prominent Oppositional Defiant Disorder symptoms include a negativistic, defiant and hostile pattern of behavior which may last for 6 months to 1 year. During this phase, the affected kid may show the following symptoms of ODD:
    - Frequent loss of temper for hardly any reason
    - Acts of violence accompanied by yelling and a destructive attitude
    - Constant argument with the adults which may get extremely irritating and frustrating for the one dealing with the affected child

- A defiant attitude and a show of refusal to abide by
- A tendency of annoying and irritating people intentionally
- Blaming others for mistakes committed by him or her and passing the bucks on to others
- Extreme touchiness and hyper sensitivity
- Getting easily annoyed and irritated by others
- An angry and resentful approach
- A vindictive & malicious attitude that at times can be very dangerous

The diagnosis of these symptoms is extremely important in Oppositional Defiant Disorder treatment. However, there are certain points that are to be kept in mind during treatment of Oppositional Defiant Disorder.

> Certain symptoms of Oppositional Defiant Disorder are the manifestation of some clinically significant impairment in regards to social, occupational or academic functioning.

> Another factor that is to be kept in mind while carrying the treatment for Oppositional Defiant Disorder is that the behaviors do not always show off solely during a Psychotic or a Mood Disorder.

> Again, if the individual in question is more than 18 years old, certain symptoms of Oppositional Defiant Disorder might not match with the ones of Conduct Disorder or Antisocial Personality Disorder.

Other associated Oppositional Defiant Disorder symptoms are:

- Problems in learning
- A depressed and frustrated mood
- Hyperactivity
- Addiction to substance
- Show of dramatic or at times antisocial personality

Differential Oppositional Defiant Disorder Diagnosis

Certain types of Oppositional Defiant Disorder may have similar or at times, exactly the same type of symptoms. Therefore, it is imperative that the doctor treating the case will have to take extra precaution to pinpoint the exact symptoms and make sure that those shown are Oppositional Defiant Disorder symptoms that he or she is intended to take care of. Following are the symptoms that may look similar in a variety of Oppositional Defiant Disorder cases

- Disorder in conduct or behavior
- Disorder in mood
- Psychotic disorder
- Attention Deficit and Hyperactivity Disorder
- Mental retardation, accompanied by occasional problem in language comprehension

Treating ODD

Oppositional Defiant Disorder is a specific type of a Disruptive Turbulent Development Disorder (DTDD) that imparts a sense of low esteem and low self confidence to children. Statistics have revealed that almost 10% of children develop these Oppositional Defiant Disorder symptoms when they grow up.

A patient with ODD symptoms has to be treated in various ways depending upon the severity of the symptoms. Let us discuss the various ways of ODD treatment.

- **Psychotherapy**:
    This is the most common treatment of patient with ODD symptoms, which can be conducted by a reputable psychotherapist who is well trained and well experienced. Apart from conducting the therapy, they are also trained to provide the family members of the patients, invaluable tips of how to behave with a child suffering from ODD and the ways of interacting with the child. They also provide tips of how to guide the child to express his or her feelings or how to cope with various situations and deal with those situations in an effective way.
- **An Effective Course of Medication**:

    This is another most effective, as well as, common form of treating ODD. The affected child can be brought to an experienced doctor who can examine the child and prescribe certain medicines that the doctor may deem applicable for the child. Generally doctors prescribe anti-psychotic drugs to the children with ODD symptoms. These drugs arrest the symptoms and reduce the ODD related problems in the patient. However, in general these drugs have a lot of side effects and as a result of this, these drugs are administered only in extreme conditions when the other process of ODD treatment the normal psychotherapy and behavioral modification methods fail to yield any positive result.

- **Behavior Modification**

This treatment method is followed in relatively moderate cases of Oppositional Defiant Disorder. In this method, the parents of a patient with ODD symptoms usually control the mental state and behavior by offering gifts and pleasantries that the child loves. Constant encouragement should be given to the affected child so as to minimize the effects of Oppositional Defiant Disorder. There are various organizations which train parents of the children who are suffering from ODD. In these organizations, various means of psychotherapy along with effective ways of treating children with Oppositional Defiant Disorder symptoms are taught to the parents so as to enable them to bring up a kid with ODD symptoms.

As Oppositional Defiant Disorder is a psychological disorder of the immature mindset of a child, it is highly imperative that upbringing of these children is done in a very careful and immaculate manner so as to reduce the symptoms of ODD before they impart any permanent damage to the psyche of the child in question. One should remember that any reluctance in the treatment process can leave irreparable damage to the child's mindset, leaving him or her mentally disoriented forever. Statistics say, the symptoms of ODD, if not taken care of properly can be inherited through generations ruining the mindset of an entire dynasty.

ODD Treatments

Handling a child or teen with oppositional defiant disorder (ODD) can be a challenging task for any parent for the simple reason that he can show disruptive behavior, throw tantrums or argue with you and others in authority. To cope up with such a child, you need the help of child development professionals, doctors and counselors along with proper treatment procedures. The treatment options for patient with ODD symptoms include therapy, medications, and social skills training.

However, before doing anything else, it's important to know whether your child is actually exhibiting any disorder symptoms. Sometimes it becomes difficult to differentiate between a child with strong emotions and will and one with oppositional defiant tendencies. Though every child shows some oppositional behavior at certain developmental age, there is always a difference in the degree of such behavior. The symptoms of ODD usually start showing before a child turns 8. In some cases, the symptoms may start reflecting little late; but these always happen before a child enters into his teens.

The signs of oppositional defiant disorder gradually develop, but these tend to get worse with passing months or years. If you see that the behavior of your child has been persistently disruptive towards home, family and school even after 6 months, you can take it as ODD sign. He can become defiant, negative, disobedient and hostile towards other authority figures. And all these may lead him to feel resentment, anger and a lack of self-esteem, throw tantrums, face performance problems in school, annoy people, argue with adults, and hold others responsible for his own misbehavior and mistakes.

Since oppositional defiant disorder can co-exist with other mental and behavioral disorders such as depression, attention deficit hyperactivity, disorder and anxiety, it becomes essential to treat the co-occurring illnesses as well. Otherwise, these can cause defiance or irritability in the child. With proper ODD treatment, you can help your child gain his self-esteem and re-establish a healthy relationship with you and family.

For treating ODD, children can be recommended different types of psychotherapy and training along with medications (if required), which have to be taken for many months or longer. The parents also need to undergo certain training. Some of these therapies and training are: parent-child interaction therapy (PCIT), social skills training, parent training, individual and family therapy, cognitive problem-solving training, etc.

With the help of most of these therapies and trainings, a child learns to deal with his anger and behavior issues and build positive and healthy relationship with his peer groups. In parent-child interaction therapy (PCIT), the therapist communicates with the child but actually gives training to his parents so that they are able to reinforce self-esteem and positive behavior in their child. Another treatment option called parent training is especially designed to help you in parenting your child with oppositional defiant disorder. With this training, you get to develop such skills which help you cope up with your ODD child with more patience and positivity and less frustration. Sometimes, your child can also become a part of this training to accomplish the desired goal together.

Remedies for ODD

ODD or Oppositional Defiant Disorder treatments can bring a difference in the life of a child who is a victim of this psychological disorder. But before going straight into the remedies, it's important to understand what Oppositional Defiant Disorder is. Oppositional Defiant Disorder (ODD) is typically found in children between 9 to 10 years of age. The signs of this kind of conduct disorders in a child are provocative behavior, defiance, and disobedience. However, a child with this ailment doesn't always show the tendency to indulge in any kind of extreme dissocial or aggressive acts which are against law or the rights of other individuals.

According to some medical experts, Oppositional Defiant Disorders in behavior are not entirely different from Conduct Disorder. However, it is difficult to find out whether the distinction between the two is quantitative or qualitative. Nonetheless, it is said that the difference between Oppositional Defiant Disorder symptoms and Conduct Disorder symptoms can only be seen in younger children. Children having Conduct Disorders show tendencies that go beyond disobedience, defiance or disruptiveness.

The main characteristics of Oppositional Defiant Disorder are negative behavior, hostility, defiance, and disruptive tendencies, etc. These patterns are not normal for a child who belongs to the same age group and has been brought up in the same socio-cultural environment. A child suffering from this disorder tends to defy the rules of the adults and irritate others intentionally. They get easily annoyed or angry by other people whom they hold responsible for their own problems or mistakes. Losing temper or becoming easily frustrated are some more signs of this mental disorder. These things seem to be more obvious when the child interacts with peers or adults in his or her acquaintances.

According to experts, talking to Oppositional Defiant Disorder patients is not easy. Parents need to learn certain techniques to communicate with their children suffering from this kind of ailment. A type of talk therapy, which is known as Cognitive-Behavioral Therapy, can be useful for both parents as well as the children. It helps in building positive thinking and is good for the whole family. In addition, certain Oppositional Defiant Disorder treatment can also be tried. Some of these are listed below.

Remedies for Oppositional Defiant Disorder

- The child should be given proper skills training to manage his or her anger and to solve problems. He or she should also be trained to be in the company of other people and to deal with strong feelings.
- Since parents need to maintain their patience while dealing with their kids with ODD, they also need to go for skills training. This will enable them to cope with problems, discipline, anger, etc. The training will impart confidence into the parents with and teach the members of the family on how to work together towards this problem. Both children as well as the parents will learn to solve problems together.
- Another part of Oppositional Defiant Disorder treatment is brining changes at home. This includes not imposing too many rules on the child in question and instead giving choices to him or her.

Creating a stringent routine and regulating leisure time for the child should also be avoided.
- Parents can also talk to the teachers at school and find out a suitable solution which can help their children cope up with their behavior problems.

Asperger's Syndrome

The Top Five Treatment Plans for Asperger's Syndrome

Asperger's Syndrome can probably best be defined as an autism spectrum ailment that is characterized by difficulties in social interaction. Since Asperger's Syndrome symptoms vary from on child to another, there is no thumb rule of treatment. However, various methods of Asperger's Syndrome treatment are carried out depending upon the age of the affected kid and the symptoms shown. At this juncture, it should be kept in mind that no medication courses are carried out for treating Asperger's Syndrome. The method of treatment is entirely dependent on the symptoms shown by the patient.

Training of Social Skills:

Children with Asperger's Syndrome often find it extremely difficult in differentiating various facial expressions and tonality of voice as and when people speak to them. This often lands them in highly embarrassing situations that make matters worse. By the social skill training, these children are taught how to differentiate between various types of facial expression and voice tonality. This will help them understand the when a person is happy or angry with them. They are also taught to understand and differentiate between jokes and sarcasm. This helps these children in socializing and mingling with people with ease and comfort.

Cognitive Conduct of Behavioral Therapy:

One of the most common Asperger's Syndrome symptoms that are noticed is the inability to gauge situations. This often lands these children in all sorts of troubled situations that make the matters increasingly embarrassing for them. Cognitive Conduct of Behavioral Therapy teaches them to gauge situation beforehand and react accordingly by applying brain and intellect. This will reduce the amount of stress they are subjected to, thereby helping them to control their temper and their overall behavior. Reduction of stress factor on their minds helps them to control their emotional outbursts, which is one most common symptoms of Asperger's Syndrome.

Parental Education:

As children are the victims of Asperger's Syndrome, it is highly important to teach parents how to deal with children who have developed Asperger's Syndrome symptoms. Improper parenting method will only make matters worse for the patients. That is why, parents of the affected children are given certain training and tips about how to children with children with Asperger's Syndrome so as to hasten the process of recovery.

Medication Course:

There are not any proper medicinal courses for patients with Asperger's Syndrome. Though therapists and psychologists prescribe certain medicines to keep the symptoms under control, majority of these medicines have adverse side effects on children. Hence, it is imperative that the patients keep a close vigil on them to make sure they are not showing any newer symptoms or there is no emergence of any side effect(s) resulting from the consumption of these medicines. Here again, parental education becomes important. Generally, these children are prescribed sleeping pills and other neurotic drugs to keep their emotions under control.

Positive Reinforcement:

This helps children suffering from Asperger's Syndrome in interacting with their parents and others in a proper way. All this processes involve a positive stance and support that imparts a sense of confidence and comfort in the patients. This helps them in taking on the society and interacting with others in a proper way in the long run.

Asperger's Syndrome Symptoms

Asperger's Syndrome (AS), which is also called Asperger's syndrome, as well as, Asperger's Disorder, is a particular variety of Autism Spectrum Disorder (ASD). This ailment is associated with certain problems in social interaction that is accompanied by certain restrictive & re repetitive behavioral patterns. The primary difference between Asperger's Syndrome and other typical ASDs is that in Asperger's Syndrome there are certain relative linguistic and cognitive developmental preservations that are not diagnosed otherwise.

Thorough research has revealed that Asperger's Syndrome is more frequent in boys than it is amongst girls. Classical symptoms of Asperger's Syndrome are generally associated with other disorders that include Tourette's disorder, depression, various kinds of attention deficit complications, and anxiety.

The following are some symptoms of Asperger's Syndrome diagnosis.

One of the main symptoms of AS that the doctors generally look for is the qualitative impairment of interpersonal interaction that involves the following characteristics:

- Impairment in the use of various non-verbal behavior that regulates the social interactions
- Inability to develop relationships that are appropriate to the age of the individual
- Inability to reciprocate socially and emotionally

Other Asperger's Syndrome symptoms that involve various kinds of restricted, stereotyped, and repetitive behavioral patterns are:

- An obsessive mindset with one or multiple typecast and restricted interest patterns
- Stubborn adherence to certain specific non-functional rituals and routines of life
- A specific stereotyped or repetitive pattern of motor mannerisms and a rigid obsession or preoccupation towards certain objects.

One of most common symptoms that are found in patients suffering from Asperger's Syndrome is their compulsive interest in certain areas, that at times amounts to an obsession. The patients, during their early childhood days generally demonstrate an obsession or in other words, an obsessive interest for a specific area or a subject. At times, their interest or obsession changes with time and the old ones are replaced by new ones. Whatever is the case, they continue to show these symptoms throughout their childhood well into their adulthood. At times, these obsessions determine the academic and professional career of these individuals. Hence, doctors diagnosing and treating Asperger's Syndrome in adults generally look for the past of these patients and try to retrieve evidence of this ailment from their childhood days.

Another extremely important symptom of Asperger's Syndrome is inability of the patients to socialize. Children who suffer from classical Autism also suffer from this symptom but they are not as impaired as the patients of Asperger's Syndrome. In fact, such is the impact of this inability that children suffering from AS cannot continue their normal lives as they are left utterly frustrated and alienated by their inability to socialize with other children.

Other common symptoms of Asperger's Syndrome include:

- Gazing at a particular object or a person too intently and evading eye contact while communicating
- Either not changing facial expression, or an exaggerated change in facial expressions
- Not using the normal comprehension of gestures while communicating
- Inability in perceiving the nonverbal cues or communicative gestures
- Inability to respect the interpersonal boundaries

PTSD

How PTSD Affects Sleep

Post-Traumatic Stress Disorder is a typical type of an anxiety disorder that is generally caused to an individual by an experience that has resulted in intense psychological trauma. Post-Traumatic Stress Disorder symptoms are generally shown by soldiers returning from battle zones after a long exposure to the violence of war and destruction. However, statistics have revealed that the effects of PTSD are not merely restricted to soldiers. Civilians (especially, children) who have met near-death situations including, abduction by terrorists and miscreants, prolonged exposure to death and destruction, mental or physical torture, and domestic violence, etc. can exhibit symptoms of Post-Traumatic Stress Disorder. Accidents and other traumatic episodes that are experienced by a child or a loved one of the child in his or her presence also results in development of Post-Traumatic Stress Disorder symptoms.

Various Post-Traumatic Stress Disorder symptoms, include disturbing memories of unpleasant episodes, sudden outbursts of emotions in the form or anger, violence of intense grief, bed wetting (especially, in cases of children). However, the most common and threatening effects of PTSD is the loss of sleep shown by children. They tend to see nightmares of the traumatic experiences whenever they try to sleep and in the process gradually develop a phobia for sleeping. This results in complete loss of sleep that complicates the condition even further.

Sleeplessness is one of the most common symptoms of most of the anxiety and stress related complications. However, in Post-Traumatic Stress Disorder, sleeplessness is the most noticeable symptom that severely interferes with the victim's sleeping habits.

A lack of sleep for a prolonged period of time increases the mental agony or any physical pain that may have been induced by the episode. The pain can be severe and turn chronic. Lack of sleep then starts affecting digestive system of the victim, by weakening the walls of the stomach. Severe or nagging headache that lasts for long is another direct effect of sleeplessness with flashbacks & thoughts recounting the traumatic episodes making the matter even worse.

Certain children with Post-Traumatic Stress Disorder symptoms even complain of hearing things and as such, are reluctant to stay alone in a room. Even, seeing certain things that apparently appear 'supernatural' are common in children with extreme Post-Traumatic Stress Disorder.

While all these are psychological problems resulted by the traumatic experience, what these children need is intense psychopathic therapy backed by proper counseling and medication that may last for months or even years depending upon the severity. Parents of these children with Post-Traumatic Stress Disorder symptoms need to take cohesive actions as well to see that they can deal with these children in a proper way and help them to overcome their trauma sooner than later.

What are some of the symptoms of PTSD?

Before we discuss the Post Traumatic Stress Disorder symptoms, it is important to know what Post Traumatic Stress Disorder is and what kind of implications it will have on an individual -

Post-Traumatic Stress Disorder or PTSD is an acute state of anxiety disorder, which may crop up after a prolonged exposure of any individual (both adult as well as children) to any incident or traumatic event that may cause extreme psychological trauma, stress and anxiety, intense fear, horror or helplessness. These incidents may range from threat of life to a serious injury to the individual or someone else whom the individual is in company with. At times certain incident(s) that may put the psychological, physical, or sexual integrity of the individual or his or her companion at stake can result in such Post Stress Disorder.

Clinically speaking, this is the fallout of an extreme case of psychological trauma and as such, it is generally less frequent than other common post traumatic stresses that people develop. Naturally, the effect of Post Stress Disorder or Post Traumatic Stress Disorder is far more enduring than anything else.

Post Traumatic Stress Disorder symptoms can be divided into the following categories. Based these symptoms, PTSD treatment is conducted by the experts.

- Intrusive Symptoms
- Avoidance Symptoms
- Arousal Symptoms

Intrusive Symptoms –

These Post Traumatic Stress Disorder symptoms include:

- Recurrent recollections of the traumatic events
- Frequent nightmares, or regular dreams of the traumatic events the individual was victim of

Avoidance Symptoms –

- Showing acute sense of anguish or agony at exposure to any event which even remotely symbolizes or resembles that incident
- Showing erratic physical response, stress and anxiety at exposure to any event which even remotely symbolizes or resembles that event
- Desperate attempts to run away from the thoughts or feeling or even discussion of the traumatic event
- Frantic efforts (that may at times extend to show of violence) to avoid the place, activities or people associated with the incident or those which may bring back memories of the experience.
- Drastic loss of interest in certain activities which were previously favorite
- A sense of detachment or separation from others

- *Arousal Symptoms*

    These Post Traumatic Stress Disorder symptoms include:

    - Irritability or sudden outbursts of violence or anger
    - A sense of Hyper vigilance and a loss of trust around everyone
    - Exaggerated startling response or petulance when called by name or touched or at sudden noises

- Trouble in sleeping or prolonged sleeping accompanied by bed wetting
- Inability of concentrating on anything
- Showing a host of other associated symptoms
- Showing no or restricted facial expressions
- A sense of frustration accompanied by a hopeless feeling in regards to future
- A terribly disturbed state of mind that may last for months
- Extremely fickle state of mind

Children who suffer from Reactive Attachment Disorder (RAD), at times, show various signs of PTSD and this proves that Post Traumatic Stress Disorder is often associated with RAD.

Parents of the children who are suffering from RAD may at times develop signs of PSTD as their prolonged effort to tackle the troubled children compel them to fall prey to various mental aberrations that may at times, result in Post Traumatic Stress Disorder.

How Natural Disasters Spark PTSD

Post-Traumatic Stress Disorder (PTSD) is a mental condition which is triggered by unpleasant or bitter life experiences. This mental health condition can develop in a person due to several factors and one of them is natural disasters which can severely damage and disrupt the lives of a considerable number of individuals. The occurrence of this ailment can be traced back to the Vietnam War at the end of which, soldiers who returned back experienced disturbing psychological symptoms and impaired functioning. Many soldiers who have returned after Gulf War and War in Afghanistan have also shown similar symptoms.

It's important to note that disasters can impact the lives of a wide range of people including both who are directly and indirectly involved in them.

Post-Traumatic Stress Disorder symptoms may differ from person to person, as per the severity of the condition and victim's experiences. Also, it's vital to point out here that the effects of PSTD may not develop immediately after the event. Rather, it can happen in an individual after a week, months or even years. Its symptoms may include flashbacks, memory issues, nightmares, relationship problems and loss of functioning. In addition to these, there can be other types of more severe symptoms as well when the individual turns violent.

The symptoms, as mentioned, can vastly vary but most of the times improve considerably with treatment. According to medical health experts, counseling and psychotherapy can be useful in treating Post-Traumatic

Stress Disorder. From this, it is easy to derive that victims of this condition do not need to live with it; they can lead an active life with proper access to help.

There are certain things which can be done as a part of Post-Traumatic Stress Disorder treatment to restore health. These include expressing feelings through any creative outlet such as art and preparation of journals, talking to a calm and caring person in order to share emotions, not ignoring the feelings associated with the traumatic event, and avoiding repetitive thinking about the dreadful event(s), etc.

It's necessary for a person suffering from Post-Traumatic Stress Disorder that he doesn't let the feeling of vulnerability and powerlessness rule his mind. He should remind himself that he can deal with difficult times with strength and skills. Also, the person needs to connect with people, instead of withdrawing himself from social life. He should try to mingle with those people who care about him. However, at the same time, it's important that other people also support him n his recovery. In this situation, behavior of the family members and friends matter a lot.

Another thing that can be done to come out of the impact of Post-Traumatic Stress Disorder is that the person should get back to his normal routine. This will help him reduce his hopelessness, anxiety and stress. He should try to regulate his timings for sleeping, eating, and relaxing. He can also set aside some time to spend with family and friends. Keeping mind occupied is essential. So, dedicating time in cooking, watching movie, and playing with kids is also a good idea.

www.ingramcontent.com/pod-product-compliance
Lightning Source LLC
Chambersburg PA
CBHW051718170526
45167CB00002B/711